Dear Mom,
Hope that you find the book interesting.
Love,
Connie

PAIN

Why Do We
Continue to Suffer?

PAIN

Why Do We
Continue to Suffer?

The Culture and Science of Pain

Connie R. Faltynek

outskirts
press

Outskirts Press, Inc.
http://www.outskirtspress.com

Paperback ISBN: 978-1-9772-1888-9
Hardback ISBN: 978-1-9772-2013-4

Library of Congress Control Number: 2019920636

Outskirts Press and the "OP" logo are trademarks belonging to Outskirts Press, Inc.

PRINTED IN THE UNITED STATES OF AMERICA

Dedicated to my husband Robert, who is my dearest love, soulmate and best friend

CONTENTS

INTRODUCTION

All of us experience pain at some point in our lives. Unfortunately, many people throughout the world suffer from unrelieved pain. Why do so many people continue to suffer? How effective are current methods to relieve pain? Are available pain-relieving methods appropriately utilized? If not, why not? Why is a person's pain often not taken seriously by others, including health care providers?

We all know what pain feels like when we stub a toe or twist an ankle. Clearly we have an injury that causes us to feel pain. Sometimes the sensation of pain can be protective, such as limiting movement of an injured limb to prevent further injury. The pain we feel when we step on a sharp object, causing us to pull away, is also a protective mechanism. But *acute* pain HURTS! In modern times, acute pain can be relieved *if* appropriate medications are provided, although this is often not the case. Why is acute pain inadequately relieved?

Chronic pain, which is pain that persists after the initial injury has healed, is different. This type of pain no longer serves a protective function and is much less understood. Medications for chronic pain are limited and they usually provide only modest relief. Chronic pain has enormous social impact, limiting the ability to work and greatly diminishing quality of life. Why is chronic pain still poorly understood and inadequately relieved?

Advances in medicine are reported almost daily. Medical and scientific journals describe new knowledge about many diseases. Television and magazines are filled with ads from pharmaceutical companies describing the value of their medications to treat a variety of human ailments. But why is unrelieved pain still a major medical problem?

The book explores these and other questions by discussing the scientific and medical reasons for inadequate pain relief, as well as the impact of culture and religion on views about pain.

Chapter 1 is a primer on pain and presents basic scientific concepts. Since I anticipate that the primary readership will be people who want to enhance their understanding about the common problem of pain but are not pain experts, I have attempted to use language accessible to the non-scientist and to avoid scientific jargon as much as possible. I realize that parts of Chapter 1 are dense, but they are included to provide background information. It is not necessary to read Chapter 1 in detail before beginning the two main sections of the book.

The book is divided into two main sections: *Historical Look at Pain and Pain Relief* and *Treatment of Pain Today*. Both sections discuss the medical science of pain and the impact of cultural/religious views on pain relief. As discussed throughout, pain has been and continues to be poorly understood, compared with many other human ailments. It is a complex sensation with both physical and emotional components. Pain is an individual's subjective experience, which in most cases cannot be objectively determined by another person, including a physician or other health care provider. Cultural and religious viewpoints can influence attitudes about pain. Christian theology in particular has debated the meaning and purpose of pain, including whether and when it should be prevented or relieved.

It is not necessary to read the chapters consecutively. Although it may be advantageous to first read Section I to gain insight into the impact of history on modern views about pain, some readers may prefer to go directly to Section II, which discusses pain and pain relief today. Chapters 5 and 6 discuss the following topics: How serious is the problem of unrelieved pain today? How good are current medications in relieving pain? Contemporary discussions about pain are often intertwined with concerns about use of prescription opioids for pain relief. As we all know, opioid abuse has reached epidemic proportions in the United States. How concerned should pain patients be about taking prescription opioids to relieve moderate or severe pain? Is the fear of opioid addiction preventing people from obtaining pain relief? Chapter 7 addresses these questions and concerns by assessing the risks and benefits of prescription opioids for pain relief. Chapter 8 describes recent research to discover better pain medications.

In addition to concerns about opioids, many people prefer to minimize their use of all pain medications and instead turn to alternative pain-relieving methods. How good are the alternative methods in relieving pain? What is known about the scientific basis for their effectiveness in relieving pain for some individuals? These questions are addressed in Chapter 9. Finally, in Chapter 10, I discuss other types of ongoing research and suggest how these studies may lead to better pain management in the future.

But pain is much more than a medical problem. Philosophers and theologians have debated the purpose and meaning of pain for millennia. Historically, pain and pain relief were often not considered to be important. Chapters 2 and 3 present historical views about pain in the Western world, especially those reflecting Christian doctrine. Pain is not unique to the human species. Chapter 4 discusses that historically, pain in other species has received little attention.

So, you may ask, why did I write this book? First of all, I have a long-standing interest in the science of pain, especially medications for pain relief. For many years, I directed research to identify new and better pain medications. I have a PhD in biochemistry and over twenty years' research experience in the fields of immunology and pain. Chapter 8 includes some of my own research experiences to discover new pain medications.

In addition to my scientific background, I became interested in learning about religious views regarding pain due to my personal background. I come from a family and culture that are deeply rooted in fundamental Christianity. This culture led my mother, who suffered from recurring major depressive episodes throughout her life, to view her illness as a punishment from God. Based on my studies about the history of pain and pain relief, I have found that Christian doctrine has often held a similar view regarding pain; i.e., pain is a punishment and therefore is to be endured without complaint. As discussed throughout the book, pain has often been misinterpreted. The same can be said about depression and also addiction.

My goal in writing is to enhance understanding about pain, including the ongoing problem of unrelieved pain, the limitations of current medications and alternative methods, as well as the impact of historical views on pain relief today. Since the primary readership will likely be a broad general audience who wish to enhance their understanding of pain, as well as health care professionals who are not pain specialists, I have attempted to present scientific topics using language accessible to non-scientists, avoiding as much scientific jargon as possible. I hope that I have succeeded in this, at least to some extent. I apologize that some parts of the book, especially

Chapter 5, contain many statistics, but I feel it necessary to document the widespread problem of unrelieved pain. Each chapter contains multiple references for those who wish to read further about a particular topic.

A central argument of the book is that both limitations of modern medicine and historical views about pain contribute to the ongoing problem of inadequate pain relief. The book emphasizes the right of people to obtain relief from unrelenting pain. I hope that the book enhances understanding about pain and, in some small way, helps to reduce pain and suffering by decreasing biases and misconceptions.

Chapter 1

WHAT *IS* PAIN? A PRIMER

Everyone experiences pain at some point, but there are many types of pain. Pain is a complex sensation, resulting from the combination of multiple biochemical, physiological, and emotional components. To begin the primer, I briefly describe various types of pain and also present basic concepts of pain transmission. The prevalence and current understanding of specific painful conditions are discussed in greater detail in Chapter 5.

TYPES OF PAIN

Although everyone knows the feeling of pain, not all pain is the same. (1, 2) Various terms have been used to describe the different types of pain. One commonly used classification is acute vs chronic pain. Acute pain is often a symptom of an underlying disease or a recent injury. In contrast, chronic pain can exist for a long time after the disease has been cured or the injury appears to have healed. In general, pain is considered chronic when it lasts longer than three months, since most injuries heal within this time period. Each of the classifications can be subdivided, as shown in Table 1.

Table 1. Classification of Major Pain Types

| **Acute Pain** |
| Nociceptive |
| Inflammatory |
| **Chronic Pain** |
| Inflammatory |
| Degenerative |
| Neuropathic |
| Fibromyalgia |

The simplest type of pain is a sub-classification of acute pain sometimes called *nociceptive pain*, meaning that we sense a noxious or unpleasant stimulus. The pain we feel when we stub our toes or hit our fingers with a hammer is acute nociceptive pain, which subsides rather quickly.

Acute nociceptive pain is an alarm signal. It is crucial for survival, since it warns of danger and causes us to pull away from the situation or object which is causing pain, thereby protecting against further injury. Some rare hereditary disorders emphasize the importance of this alarm signal. Individuals with these disorders do not feel pain and, as a result, frequently injure themselves because they do not have the protection provided by the sensation of pain. (3, 4)

But even when the pain warning system is intact, tissue injury often occurs. The body then tries to heal the injury by calling for help from the inflammatory system. Inflammation occurs when specific types of cells and certain molecules, known as inflammatory mediators, are recruited to the site of injury. Inflammatory cells and mediators aid the healing process, but they also produce the type of pain known as inflammatory pain.

As with nociceptive pain, *inflammatory pain* also serves a protective function, but in a different way. Inflammation produces heightened sensitivity to stimuli. Mild stimuli that normally do not cause pain become painful after injury. More intense stimuli that usually cause only minor pain produce more severe pain (Figure 1). As a result, an individual with inflammatory pain will try to protect the injured area to limit the pain and therefore may prevent further injury.

Inflammatory pain usually lasts only a relatively short time, ranging from hours to a few days. But under some conditions, inflammatory pain can persist for a long time and become chronic. Chronic inflammatory diseases which have pain as a symptom include rheumatoid arthritis and inflammatory bowel disease.

Chronic pain also occurs with some degenerative conditions, such as osteoarthritis (OA). Especially in the early stages of OA, there is associated inflammation, but pain can persist after the inflammation has resolved. Degeneration of cartilage in the joints is the major cause of OA and its associated chronic pain. Cartilage, which is a slippery tissue between the ends of bone, normally enables smooth movement of bones. But when the cartilage degenerates, the characteristic symptoms of OA, such as pain and stiffness, occur.

A nerve injury which does not readily repair itself can also lead to chronic pain. This type of pain is called *neuropathic pain*. There is no known protective purpose for neuropathic pain, but rather it is considered a dysfunction. As in inflammatory pain, a nerve injury can cause pain in response to stimuli that normally are not painful and more severe pain in response to stimuli that are usually only mildly painful (Figure 1). Neuropathic pain can be

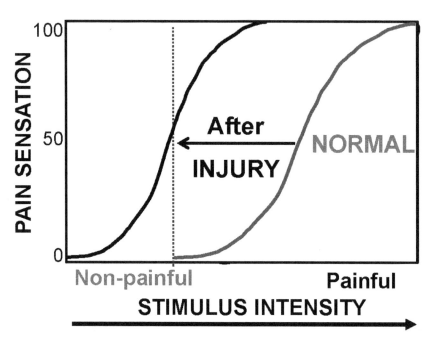

Figure 1. Injury Increases Pain Sensation

The level of pain is indicated in arbitrary values from 0 to 100 on the y-axis. The intensity of a stimulus is indicated on the x-axis going from left to right. The stimulus can vary from a very minor one which is normally not painful to a very strong stimulus which does evoke pain. After an injury, due to inflammation or nerve damage, the same types of stimuli cause greater pain. For example, lightly touching the skin with clothing is normally not painful, but can cause severe pain in patients with neuropathic pain. Similarly, touching one's hand with a hot iron normally evokes a moderate level of pain, but the pain is greater if the iron touches an area that has tissue damage from a previous injury.

excruciating. Even loose clothing which only gently touches the skin can cause severe pain. Neuropathic pain can also be spontaneous, occurring without any type of stimulus. Patients with neuropathic pain often describe the pain as burning, shooting, tingling, or like an electric shock. Neuropathic pain is still poorly understood. Medications usually provide only modest relief. This type of pain is the result of multiple changes in the nervous system which occur after the initial nerve injury. One common type of neuropathic pain often develops in people with uncontrolled diabetes. Several other disorders, including multiple sclerosis, can also lead to neuropathic pain.

Fibromyalgia is another type of chronic pain. It has been widely misunderstood in the past. Current understanding of fibromyalgia is discussed in Chapter 5.

There are other types of pain which don't fit easily into any of the categories in Table 1. For example, the pain of migraine is a complex disorder involving both the nervous and the vascular systems. In addition to the pain, there are other disabling symptoms including nausea, vomiting, extreme sensitivity to sound or light. Most sufferers have attacks once or twice a month, although for some people migraine is a chronic illness with at least fifteen migraine days a month. (5) The major physiological basis of migraine is still hotly debated. (6)

MECHANISMS OF PAIN TRANSMISSION

In the 17th century, René Descartes depicted acute nociceptive pain in a drawing which has been included in many medical textbooks ever since. In this famous drawing, activation of nerves in the foot sends a signal through the spinal cord to the brain, much as pulling a rope causes the bell to ring in a church tower (Figure 2). It is important to note that we actually feel pain only after the nerve impulse reaches the brain. The Descartes drawing made in the 17th century is still basically accurate today, although we now know that pain transmission is much more complex than in this early depiction.

To start the discussion of current understanding of pain transmission, let's begin by describing normal sensations which may

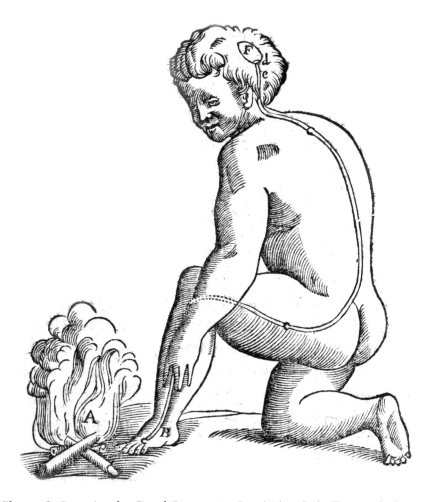

Figure 2. Drawing by René Descartes Depicting Pain Transmission.
Published in 1677 by Amstelodami: Danielem Elsevirium.

or may not be painful. As shown in Figure 3, different types of
nerves are activated in the periphery under different conditions
to generate either a non-painful sensation or a relatively low level of pain. A light touch, such as stroking the skin with a feather,
activates low- threshold nerve fibers. These nerve fibers, known
as Aβ fibers, give rise to a non-painful sensation. In contrast,

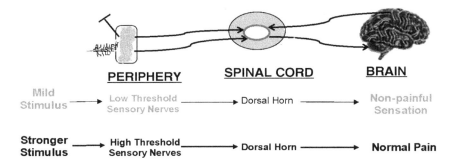

Figure 3. Normal Sensations

A mild stimulus, such as a feather brushing the skin, activates nerves on the skin. A stronger stimulus, such as stepping on a tack, activates different nerves which have a higher threshold for activation. Both types of nerves relay the information to a region in the spinal cord known as the dorsal horn, and then up to the brain. It is the brain which interprets the incoming signal as either a painful or non-painful sensation.

a stronger stimulus, such as a cutting a finger with a knife or stepping on a small sharp object, activates high-threshold nerve fibers, called Aδ and C fibers, generating pain (Figure 3). If there is no significant tissue or nerve damage, this type of pain, which quickly subsides, is *normal pain* or acute nociceptive pain.

However, after a more significant injury which did damage tissues or nerves, the pain can be considered *pathological pain*. This type of pain is no longer simply a warning of danger, but it is a signal that something actually is wrong. Due to the damage, nerves in the periphery and/or the spinal cord become sensitized, i.e., have heightened sensitivity and are on high alert (Figure 4). As a result, even mild stimuli can cause pain, and more intense stimuli produce even greater pain (Figures 1 and 4).

Moreover, when peripheral nerves are continuously bombarded with a painful stimulus, the pain often gets worse. This has

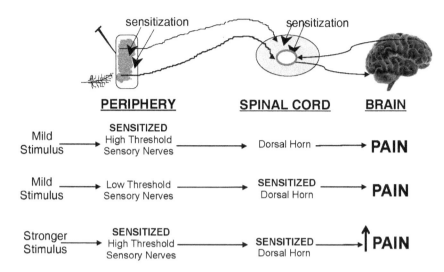

Figure 4. Pathological Pain

Pathological pain, which occurs after an injury, happens when nerves in the periphery or in the spinal cord become sensitized due to the presence of certain natural chemicals (neurotransmitters) released after injury. As a result, even mild stimuli now cause pain and stronger stimuli cause greater pain.

been shown in experimental studies, in which volunteer individuals rated the level of pain caused by very short applications of a heat stimulus. Pain was rated using the Visual Analog Scale (VAS), in which 0 means no pain, whereas 100 is the worst pain imaginable. (7) After a single short application of heat, the individuals rated their pain as low; i.e., <20 on the pain scale. However, after repeated applications of the same temperature at 3 second intervals, pain levels became severe, reaching >80 on the VAS scale, as shown in Table 2.

Table 2. Repeated painful stimuli increase pain severity

Number of Successive Stimuli	Pain Rating (VAS)
1	12
3	25
5	46
7	65
10	80
15	88

[Adapted from Reference 7; Figure 3]

The more severe pain, which occurred after repeated stimuli, is much more than an interesting experimental observation. Rather, it enhances understanding how acute pain that is initially rather mild can become more severe or even develop into chronic pain. The demonstration that a non-painful or mildly painful stimulus becomes more painful with repeated applications argues that acute pain should be aggressively managed to prevent the pain from getting worse. Even after the actual cause of the pain is removed, the nerves continue to send pain signals due to several neurological and biochemical processes that have been set in motion.

Figures 3 and 4 schematize how the pain signal is sent from peripheral nerves to the spinal cord and then to the brain. We feel pain only after the signal reaches the brain. A variety of mechanisms are involved in this pathway, starting at the surface of peripheral nerves. A somewhat simplified diagram of the cell membrane at the surface of a neuron is shown in Figure 5. Peripheral nerves contain many types of cell surface receptors that are specific for different stimuli. One of these receptors is an ion channel known as TRPV1, which is discussed in detail in Chapter 8. TRPV1 is a major sensor for heat, which is the stimulus used in the experimental pain study described above. TRPV1 can also be activated by several other stimuli to generate pain (Figure 5).

The surface of peripheral nerves also contains receptors for other molecules which modify neuronal activity and play a role in pain transmission. They include receptors for the prostaglandins discussed in Chapter 6 and nerve growth factor (NGF) discussed in Chapter 8. Receptors for these important molecules are also shown in Figure 5.

After the cell surface receptors are activated, signals are sent to the inside of the cell, in this case the neuron. These signals can be biochemical or "electrical." Both types of signals occur in neurons, but electrical signals are especially important. All cells

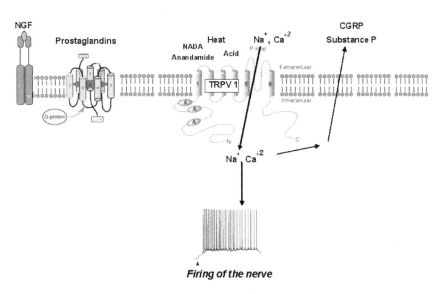

Figure 5. Multiple Mechanisms Can Activate Peripheral Nerves

The cell surface of peripheral nerves contains receptors for many types of pain-inducing molecules. After these molecules bind to their receptors, a variety of events occur inside the cell, leading to firing of the nerve and release of neurotransmitters, such as CGRP and substance P, which propagate the pain signal to other nerves.

maintain a difference in ion concentrations between outside and inside of the cells. Neurons are known as *excitatory cells*, meaning that when certain ions enter the cell through an open channel, the electrical potential changes across the cell membrane. This results in membrane depolarization and a process known as action potential firing (Figure 5). The firing is then propagated to other nearby neurons.

The surface of neurons contains several types of ion channels which regulate the concentrations of ions inside the cells. TRPV1 in Figure 5 is one type of ion channel. When activated, TRPV1 changes its conformation, which opens the channel, allowing both sodium ($Na+$) and calcium ($Ca++$) ions to enter the neuron. Increases in $Na+$ ions cause the neuron to *fire,* whereas increases in $Ca++$ ions alter many biochemical events inside the cells. Subsequently, molecules known as *neurotransmitters*, such as substance P and CGRP, are released from terminals of the neuron (Figure 5). The neurotransmitters then bind to the surface of adjacent neurons, thereby transmitting the excitation to other neurons. Some of the neurotransmitters which facilitate pain transmission are listed in Table 3. Repeated stimulation of peripheral nerves increases the release of some of these molecules, increasing the level of pain.

Table 3. Naturally Occurring Molecules Which Either Increase or Decrease Pain

Neurotransmitters Which Increase Pain	Neurotransmitters Which Decrease Pain
Substance P Calcitonin gene-related peptide (CGRP) Glutamate Bradykinin	Norepinephrine Serotonin γ-aminobutyric acid (GABA) Endorphins

However, the sensation of pain is even more complex than transmitting pain signals between neurons and ultimately from the site of injury to the brain. In addition to the pathway that transmits the pain signal up to the brain, the brain sends signals back to the spinal cord to modulate the sensation of pain, as schematized in Figures 3 and 4.

There are two types of neurotransmitters. Some convey the pain signal from peripheral nerves to the brain, thereby generating pain, whereas others blunt pain sensation (Table 3). These molecules, which either increase or decrease pain sensation, are part of a control mechanism consisting of opposing physiological systems. This type of control is not unique to pain. All physiological systems are regulated through checks and balances. Some mechanisms generate one effect, whereas competing mechanisms cause the opposite effect. Indeed, the human body has multiple systems which must remain in balance to remain healthy. This is known as *homeostasis,* from the Greek words roughly translated as similar (homeo) to the state of equilibrium between opposing equal forces (stasis).

Without these checks and balances, life as we know it would not be possible. For an analogy, consider the disastrous results if a car had only an accelerator, without a brake to slow it down. Similarly, a physiologic system without control would quickly run amok. Not only is it necessary to have opposing physiological mechanisms, but they must remain in balance to maintain health. Indeed, many diseases are caused by an imbalance in opposing systems. One example is diabetes. Normally, our bodies make appropriate amounts of both insulin, which decreases the level of glucose in circulation, and glucagon, which increases the glucose level. In diabetes, insulin either is not produced in adequate amounts or is no longer able to function appropriately, causing an imbalance in the normal systems regulating glucose levels. Consistently high glucose levels lead to the severe complications of uncontrolled diabetes.

Similarly, chronic pain can be characterized as an imbalance in regulatory systems and even has been called a disease in itself, rather than simply a symptom. (8) The imbalance that exists in chronic pain may be due to ongoing excessive neuronal input from the periphery to the brain and/or inadequate output from the brain back to the spinal cord. There is evidence that the normal inhibitory signals from the brain back to the spinal cord are deficient in some chronic pain patients. (9) This appears to be the case in the chronic pain characteristic of fibromyalgia. (10-12)

PAIN: IT *IS* ALL IN YOUR HEAD!

As discussed in other chapters, chronic pain has often been dismissed as being "all in the patient's head." This derogatory statement is sometimes made when no underlying physical cause can be identified for the pain. As commonly understood, this means that the patient is simply imagining the pain.

But interpreting the phrase literally, indeed all pain *is* in your head. The sensation of pain occurs only when the brain integrates and interprets the various incoming signals. Multiple regions of the brain are involved in the sensation of pain. These include the periaqueductal grey in the brainstem, which receives the incoming signals from the periphery via the spinal cord; the thalamus, which relays the signals to the higher levels of consciousness in the cerebral cortex; and the limbic system, which governs emotions. (13)

IMPACT OF EMOTIONS AND THOUGHTS ON PAIN SENSATION

As discussed in Chapter 2, the ancients considered pain to be only an *emotion*, not a physical sensation. But we now know that pain is the result of defined physical processes. Nevertheless, we also know that a person's emotional state and thoughts can affect the physical sensation of pain.

One example of the effect of a person's thoughts on the perception of pain is the *placebo effect*. This occurs when an individual reports feeling less pain, even though he had received a dummy sugar pill but thought he had received a pain-relieving medication (see Chapter 9). Another example of the effect of an individual's thoughts and emotions on pain sensation often occurs with patient-controlled analgesia (PCA). Today it is common for hospitalized patients to use PCA to control the amount of opioid medications they receive. Interestingly, patients who use PCA often report less pain, even though they are receiving the same amount of medication as patients who received their opioids directly from a clinician. (14-16) It is well known that anxiety increases the perceived level of pain. PCA provides patients with a sense of control over their pain, thereby reducing their anxiety and decreasing the perceived pain level. Some studies have shown that patients receiving their opioid medication by PCA experienced not only less pain, but also less sedation. (15) Since sedation is a common side effect of opioids, the lower level of sedation confirms that the patients had indeed obtained pain relief with less medication. Clearly the mind; i.e., the brain, is at work in the perception of pain! *All pain is in your head,* since the brain integrates sensations from physical stimuli with emotions and thoughts to generate an individual's overall pain perception. (17, 18)

Western world philosophies typically view the human mind and body as distinct and separate entities. Medicine is the science of the body, whereas psychology is the science of the mind. The body is considered to be anatomical and physiological, whereas the mind is the seat of emotions and thoughts. As a result, most discussions about pain have been divided into the two compartments of body and mind; i.e., physical and psychological. The concept of the body is readily understood as a physical entity.

But what exactly is the mind? Most people agree that thoughts and emotions are centered in the brain, although the mind is still mysterious due to the poorly understood complexities of the brain. However, as knowledge about the brain increases, it is my belief as a scientist that eventually the brain will be considered simply another bodily organ which functions through defined physical mechanisms. I would argue that as knowledge about the brain increases, the artificial distinction between mind and body in relation to pain will diminish. The mind and emotions that constitute the psychological aspects of pain will no longer be viewed as mysterious entities, but rather the result of intricate biochemistry in the brain. The current division between the psychological and physical aspects of pain will become unified. Any other concept is beyond science and remains in the realm of mystery and religion.

CONCLUSION

There are many types of pain, but all involve transmission of information from a painful stimulus to the brain. Multiple physiological and biochemical mechanisms are involved in pain transmission, including those which enhance pain and those which can diminish pain. Emotions and thoughts can deeply affect an individual's pain perception. Although our knowledge of pain has substantially increased in recent years, there is still much we don't understand. No doubt, future research will enhance our understanding about the complexities of pain transmission and perception.

SECTION I

HISTORICAL LOOK AT PAIN AND PAIN RELIEF

CHAPTER 2

⸺✦⸺

PAIN AND PAIN RELIEF PRIOR TO THE 19TH CENTURY

The history of pain is an integral part of the history of Western philosophy and religion. At various times, pain has been considered a blessing, a punishment, or simply something to be ignored. It has sometimes taken on mysterious connotations, especially when it continues long after an original injury has healed. In the past, pain has even been attributed to supernatural causes or to the presence of demons. Even today, when no cause can be identified, pain is sometimes not considered "real medical pain," but rather a psychological or psychiatric disorder. In this chapter I discuss historical viewpoints about pain in the Western world, from antiquity up to the 19th century.

PAIN IN THE ANCIENT WESTERN WORLD

The ancient Greeks and Romans did not believe that pain served any positive purpose. Perhaps some physicians at this time did view pain as a symptom for an underlying disease. But more often, both physicians and philosophers thought that pain was simply a disorder which should be avoided or ignored.

The Greek philosopher Aristotle lived in the 4th century BCE. Aristotle, like his teacher Plato, initially viewed pain not as a sensation but as an emotion. (1) According to Aristotle, the negative emotion of pain occurred when evil spirits entered the body through an injury. (2) Later, he espoused that all knowledge and emotions were based on perception and that pain was the perception of something contrary: *"dolor est sensus rei contrariae"*. (3) Aristotle thought that conditions which caused pain, such as illness and injury, should be avoided and cured as much as possible, but he did not necessarily consider that pain *per se* should be relieved.

The philosophy of Stoicism, which was founded by Zeno in the 3rd Century BCE, was popular in the Roman Empire. It provided a guide to life on earth, without concern for an afterlife. The Stoics of antiquity did not deny the existence of pain, but rather maintained that pain was not important enough to disturb the overall well-being of a rational person. (4)

Thus, philosophers in ancient Greece did not consider pain to be of great importance in human existence. To Aristotle and the Platonists, it was the cause of pain, not pain itself that was to be avoided. To the Stoics, pain should simply be dismissed.

The Roman emperor Marcus Aurelius, who is widely regarded as epitomizing the practice of Stoic philosophy, wrote a treatise entitled *Meditations* in 170-180 CE as a guide for his own self-improvement. He wrote in this treatise that "If you suffer pain because of some external cause, what troubles you is not the thing but your decision about it, and this is in your power to wipe out at once." (5) To paraphrase, a person can abolish any suffering from pain simply through his own will power. The logical extension of this view is that an individual is responsible for his own suffering by allowing pain to be perceived, and therefore the individual can be *blamed* for his suffering. Marcus Aurelius goes on to say "Whosoever therefore is not himself indifferent to pain..., which Universal Nature employs indifferently, plainly commits sin." (6) The idea that an individual is personally responsible for suffering from pain has continued into the modern age, as discussed later in this chapter and the following chapter.

But most people through the ages likely wanted their pain to be relieved through use of any existing external remedies. Many pain-relieving remedies, which were primarily extracts derived from plants, were known in the ancient Western world. The most detailed lists of pain-relieving extracts used in the ancient world were recorded by Pliny (*Naturalis Historia*), Celsus (*De Medicina*) and Dioscorides (*De Materia Medica*) in the 1st century CE. (7, 8)

Extracts from poppies (*Papaver somniferum*) were likely the most common medicines used by the ancients to alleviate pain. Pliny described detailed methods to prepare poppy extracts, which were applied to the skin to alleviate pain in the joints or taken internally dissolved in milk to reduce other types of pain or to induce sleep. He called the extracts "opium." The emphasis Pliny placed on preparing "medication" for relieving pain suggests that he believed pain should be actively eliminated using the available methods. (8)

Use of poppy extracts to relieve pain predated the description by Pliny in the 1st century CE. Archeologists have obtained evidence for poppy extracts as early as the fourth millennium BCE. (9) The earliest written reference to the use of poppies to relieve pain is considered to be the Ebers Papyrus from 1552 BCE, which in the English translation says: "The goddess Isis gave the juice of the poppy to Ra, the sun god, to treat his headache." (10)

The ancients also used opium to either induce a feeling of well-being or cause sedation. Homer wrote in *The Odyssey* in 800 BCE about Telemachus, who, when visiting Menelaus in Sparta, was overcome by sadness when he thought of all the warriors killed in the Trojan War. Helen, the daughter of Zeus, added "nepenthe", an opium preparation, to the wine served to Telemachus and other guests at the banquet so that they might forget all the evils that had occurred. (9)

So, the ancient world knew that opium could relieve physical pain, but also could relieve various types of psychological pain through its psychoactive effects. By the 1st century CE, Pliny wrote not only about the usefulness of opium, but also the dangers. (8) Today, abuse of opioids is clearly a major issue, especially in the United States. Current controversies about opioid use for pain relief are discussed extensively in Chapter 7.

PAIN IN THE EARLY CHRISTIAN ERA

In the early Christian era, physical pain took on greater significance. Pain was considered to be an inevitable part of human existence. Christian narratives frequently described humans as physical bodies in pain and emphasized the considerable suffering of mankind. The historian Judith Perkins pointed out that these representations were quite different from the prevailing traditional Greco-Roman views that the soul/mind controlled the body and therefore pain should not cause great suffering. (11) Instead, Christianity emphasized the physical pain and suffering of mankind.

This emphasis on human pain and suffering reflects the modern Christian teaching that Jesus Christ as a human experienced pain and suffering during his crucifixion. However, great theological debates took place in the early Christian Church, often about the nature of Jesus Christ. Was he always divine or was he also a human, who felt pain like the rest of us, during his time on earth? Some early Christian writings, such as the non-canonical Synoptic Gospel of Saint Peter written in the 2nd century, stated that Christ was always divine and did *not* appear to feel or to suffer from human pain during his crucifixion. (12) These writings were later declared heresies, resulting in the exclusion of the Gospel of St. Peter from the current Christian New Testament.

Jesus' earthly pain and suffering became an important part of Christian doctrine and played a substantial role in the spread of Christianity. (13) The universality of pain and the connections people felt to the suffering of Jesus are considered to have contributed to the success of Christianity in achieving both social and political power. (11)

The Christian view of pain continued to evolve as the new religion spread across the Roman Empire. A new concept began to emerge. The Christian church began to teach that human pain and suffering could have a *positive* purpose. St. Augustine of Hippo (354-430) believed that certain modes of suffering could lead to moral improvement. He urged concern for suffering individuals but did not suggest that all pain and suffering should be eliminated. (14, 15)

The doctrine of the Catholic Church in the 6th century continued to reflect dichotomy regarding pain; i.e., Christians should express empathy towards others who were suffering but also accept that pain can serve a divine purpose. Pope Gregory I, who reigned from 590 – 604, wrote extensively about the value of physical pain. He wrote that pain might serve a redemptive purpose, since it could lead to fear and contemplation, and therefore virtue. Pain was a means to encourage people to forgo worldly pleasures and instead to focus on the blessed afterlife. Although Pope Gregory taught that pain was morally uplifting and served a positive purpose, when he was personally suffering, he wrote in public letters that he wanted *his* pain to go away. (16)

PAIN IN THE MIDDLE AGES

By the 5th century, Christ's human suffering had become part of Christian orthodoxy. Nevertheless, prior to the 11th century,

Christ was usually portrayed in art as a majestic ruler, rather than as someone suffering on the cross. It was a few centuries later that the modern image of a suffering Christ on the cross became widespread in both high and low culture. In the Middle Ages, images of the suffering of Christ during his crucifixion began to exert significant effects on people's attitudes towards their own pain. (13)

The belief that pain was positive because it was morally uplifting continued to expand within the Christian world. In this era, pain was even to be welcomed, as indicated by the phrase *de bono doloris* (the good pain). As the historian Esther Cohen wrote: "Illness, misfortune, penitence, and punishment could bring salvation precisely because they were painful." (17) She further wrote that the 13th century Bishop of Paris, William of Auvergne, considered that "Pain is a God-given medicine to cure human souls, granted out of the Creator's goodness. Any...attempt to circumvent it means refusing the remedy for the ill." (18) The Dominican friar Johannes Herolt, who died in 1468, viewed pain as *imitatio Christi,* thereby providing dignity and some consolation to those who were suffering. (19) According to Cohen, Johannes Herolt said in a sermon that "All sickness...was a harbinger of death sent by Christ to encourage people to prepare for leaving the world." (19) Herolt believed that sickness and pain helped people concentrate on the health of the soul. (20)

Most people were not healthy during the Middle Ages. The lives of the vast majority of people were characterized by illness, pain, and great suffering. In the midst of such suffering, the clergy and hierarchy of the Catholic Church probably felt impotent. Perhaps the Church began to attribute a higher purpose to pain, so that people would suffer less if they believed that their pain was a gift from God to provide a path to salvation.

Theological debates among Christians continued in the Middle Ages. Philosophers and theologians began to question the meaning of pain. How could they reconcile suffering with a merciful omnipo-tent God? Why should God allow *good people* to suffer? Perhaps the Church of the Middle Ages considered that the way to reconcile human pain with a merciful omnipotent God was to attribute a di-vine purpose to pain and suffering.

Along with the view in the Middle Ages that pain was a *gift* from God to help people attain salvation, a different view also ex-isted: i.e., pain was a *punishment* from God. Christianity taught that the fall of Adam and Eve from grace, as described in the Book of Genesis in the Old Testament, caused God to punish mankind by allowing pain and suffering. But if pain given by God as punishment led to penitence and salvation, pain could also become a blessing. In addition to the view at this time that pain due to illness had a divine purpose, which could be either a gift or a punishment, some monastic orders believed that self-invoked physical pain might ex-punge sin. Examples included the wearing of hairshirts and the flag-ellation that occurred in some medieval monasteries. (20)

Therefore, a distinct paradox existed in the Middle Ages. Despite the ubiquitous message from the Catholic Church that pain was morally beneficial, it is likely that most people simply wanted to reduce their pain and suffering.

The statement by William of Auvergne, quoted above, suggests that he considered physicians who tried to relieve pain were acting contrary to God's will. But what about physicians themselves in the medieval era? Did they believe that pain was a positive force, as taught by the Church, or did they attempt to alleviate the pain of their patients?

Physicians at medieval universities did, indeed, teach and prac-tice pain relief. Medical texts of this era described methods to al-leviate pain. Based on her study of medical textbooks from the late Middle Ages, the historian Esther Cohen wrote that she was "un-able to find any procedure or medication that was recommended

because it was painful." (21) Other historical texts indicate that physicians in the Middle Ages used the limited methods available to
alleviate pain, despite the Church's view that pain had a positive
influence. The medical community considered pain to be inevitable
but not something to seek or value. (22)

PAIN IN THE 16TH, 17TH, AND 18TH CENTURIES

By the 16th century, the suffering and pain of Christ had become
important doctrines of the Christian church and were considered
essential to the sacrifice by Christ. People connected to Christ via
the shared sensation of pain. The view that unsolicited pain should
be equated with the suffering of Christ continued to spread. (13)

This was also the time of mystical saints. Christian mysticism
dealt with the relation of physical pain to spiritual transformation.
This transformation included ecstatic experiences, which involved
mystical suffering that caused visible physical bruises and wounds.
Similarly, some later martyrs were made saints not because of their
suffering, but because of a miracle which apparently enabled them
not to feel pain. (12)

Saint Teresa of Avila (1515-1582) and Saint John of the Cross
(1542-1591) were Spanish Carmelite mystics in the 16th century
who founded the Discalced Carmelite order. (23, 24) The Catholic
Church emphasized that Saint Teresa's life centered around imi-
tation of the life and suffering of Jesus. But Saint Teresa herself
described that her suffering was "in itself blissful." The motto associated with her is "To die, Lord, or to suffer! I ask nothing else of
Thee for myself but this!" (25) It is the ecstasy of Saint Teresa, not
suffering, that is usually portrayed in painting and sculpture from
this era. One author wrote the following about Saint Teresa: "The
pain she felt was not caused by mortification nor by remorse." It
was not atonement or purge of her sins, but rather her pain "forged
an organic unity with the bliss caused by her visions of Heaven."

(25) Similarly, the French Catholic nun and mystic, Saint Marguerite Maria Alacoque (1647-1690) stated, "Nothing but pain makes my life supportable." (26)

The Catholic Church in the 16th and 17th centuries continued to preach that human pain had value because it could be morally uplifting. But these were also times of great upheaval in the Church. The Protestant Reformation, occurring at this time, denounced the doctrines that humans could take part in the sufferings of Jesus Christ and that pain and suffering provided ways to salvation. As such, the Reformation attempted to take away one of the most powerful tenets of the Roman Catholic Church. In response, the Counter Reformation placed even greater emphasis on the value of physical suffering, as had characterized the doctrine of late medieval Catholicism. The theological meaning of pain was, accordingly, central to the power struggle for religious authority in this era. (27)

Medicine advanced significantly in the 17th century as knowledge of anatomy and physiology increased. For example, William Harvey published the modern understanding of the circulation of blood in 1628. The French philosopher, mathematician, and scientist René Descartes (1596-1650) developed the first mechanistic understanding of the phenomenon of pain. His theoretical diagram of pain transmission shown in Chapter 1 is still widely used in textbooks today.

Thomas Sydenham (1624-1689) is often called the father of English medicine. He considered that pain relief, not pain itself, was God-given. (28) Sydenham developed a preparation called laudanum, which consisted of opium, wine, saffron, cinnamon, and cloves. It was used not only to relieve pain, but also to promote sleep and to treat dysentery, diseases of the nervous system, and multiple other ailments. Use of laudanum became widespread in Protestant England, but less so in conservative Catholic France. (29) Sydenham was a strong champion of the use of opium in laudanum and stated: "I cannot but break out in praise of the great God, the Giver of all good things, who hath granted to the human race, as a comfort in their afflictions, no medicine of the value of opium....So necessary an instrument is opium in the hand of a skillful man, that medicine would be a cripple without it; and whoever understands it well, will do more with it alone than he could well hope to do from any single medicine." (29, 30)

Although the Catholic Church still considered that pain could have a positive, ennobling effect, a growing number of people believed that it was appropriate for a Christian to perform or receive medical relief of pain. As a result, conflicts grew in the 17th century between the Church and medicine regarding the purpose and meaning of pain. (31)

By the 18th century, which is often called the Age of Enlightenment, philosophers and physicians/scientists increasingly separated religion and philosophy from science. Pain came to be viewed as a medical and physiological problem, distinct and totally separate from concepts of salvation or punishment. (32) Pain was routinely treated using opium and laudanum in the 18th century, since most physicians at this time did not think that opium was any more dangerous than other available potions and medications. Still, there were some at this time who thought that pain was beneficial, but from a medical rather than the earlier religious perspective. For example, pain following surgery was considered to indicate that healing was occurring. Use of sedatives was believed to lower the success rate of surgery. (32)

In the 18th century, still another view about pain emerged. As historian Roselyn Rey wrote: "Bodily pain was interpreted as a sign that the soul was suffering." (33) Some types of physical pain were attributed to psychological conflicts. Pain and mental illnesses began to be considered together. The view that a patient had personal responsibility for his pain or mental illness harkened back to an extension of ancient Stoicism which appeared to blame the individual for his suffering. This was not the medieval idea that pain or mental disorders were punishments from God for wrongdoing, but rather that they could be simply controlled through stronger personal character or religious faith. This view continued in the 19th and 20th centuries, as discussed in the next chapter.

HISTORICAL VIEWS ABOUT PAIN IN THE MUSLIM AND JEWISH WORLDS

Although historical views about pain discussed thus far have primarily focused on the Christian world, it is useful to briefly draw some comparisons with views in the Muslim and Jewish worlds. Some basic religious beliefs, which differ between those of Christianity and those of Islam and Judaism, have influenced the philosophies and theological debates about human pain. The Christian Church teaches that Christ was both the Son of God and a human who suffered pain. In contrast, Judaism and Islam view the prophets as only human; God and humans are strictly separate. As a result, the meaning of pain has *not* been a subject of intense theological debate in Judaism and Islam, as it has been for centuries in Christianity. (34)

The Muslim world was the center of intellectualism during the Dark Ages in Western Europe. Avicenna (born in 980 CE) was a renowned intellectual from Persia who published extensively on a wide range of topics. He considered pain to be a *non-natural* state, imposed on the human body. This concept was quite different from the prevailing Christian view which considered pain to be punishment from God and an integral part of the *natural* state of mankind after the fall of Adam and Eve. (35) The latter view persisted for millennia in the Christian world and it significantly hindered the development of medicine, including ways to relieve pain.

In contrast, medicine advanced in the Arab world, as physicians and scholars searched for physical causes and treatments for pain.

As Thomas Dormandy wrote, referring to Avicenna's philosophy and ideas of medicine in the Dark Ages, "Islamic doctors were encouraged to believe that Allah created no ailment without creating a remedy for it, even if it was beyond the wit of man to discover what the remedy was." (36)

Avicenna's writings had wide-ranging influence in the Arab world and subsequently in the Christian world following translations of the texts into Latin. One of his major works, the *Canon of Medicine*, was translated from the Arabic into Latin by Gerard of Cremona in the 12th century. This Latin translation was a standard medical text for centuries at many universities. (35) Unfortunately, Arab medicine declined after 1300 when the Ottoman Turks became the dominant Muslim power and showed little interest in science. (36)

Christianity teaches that God is and always has been good and omnipotent. Consequently, Christians often ask: why does evil exist and why do innocent people suffer from illness and pain? Jon Levenson, Professor of Jewish Studies at Harvard University, wrote that the Jewish answer is that "the world is not yet at that stage in which God's will is absolute and unchallenged. Reality has not yet gotten to the point when the universe is simply governed by a good, omniscient, omnipotent and unchallenged deity." He goes on to describe the Jewish view by stating: "the world is not currently governed by a deity who has actualized all his potentialities and thus blasted evil and the suffering it produces from his world. And yet that deity has solemnly pledged that such a world will come into existence and has given human beings a key role in bringing that future about." (37) I paraphrase Levenson's statements as follows: Judaism considers the world to be a work in progress towards a day when good will triumph and evil will be banished. (37, 38) By extrapolation, I suggest this means that we should not puzzle about the current existence and meaning of pain and suffering, since the world is still moving toward the time when pain and suffering will no longer exist. Also writing about the Jewish viewpoint, Esther Benbassa further stated: "The problem in Scripture does not consist in determining *why* suffering exists, but in learning the reasons for the unfair way it which it is distributed." [italicization is mine] (39)

CONCLUSION

Ancient philosophers, especially the Stoics, wrote that physical pain should not cause great suffering and could be alleviated through personal will power. Nevertheless, there is considerable evidence that opium was used in the ancient Western world to relieve pain.

With the rise of Christianity, pain took on theological significance. The earthly pain and suffering of Jesus became an important doctrine of Christianity. Human pain was considered to be a blessing from God, since it could bring people closer to God, but it could also be a punishment for those who had sinned. As medical science advanced in the 17th century, conflicts grew between Christian theological views about pain and the ability of medicine to relieve pain. As will be discussed in the next chapter, new developments in pain prevention and relief were not always widely embraced in Christianity.

This chapter concludes with a brief discussion that, in contrast with Christianity, pain did not take on great theological significance in the Muslim and Jewish faiths. Since the book is focused primarily on pain in the Western World, it is beyond the scope of this book to discuss other major religions, such as Buddhism and Hinduism, which originated and are primarily practiced in the Eastern World.

CHAPTER 3

PAIN AND PAIN RELIEF IN THE 19ᵀᴴ AND 20ᵀᴴ CENTURIES

Significant medical advances to relieve pain, including the discovery of anesthesia and the birth of the hospice movement, occurred during the 19th and 20th centuries. Nevertheless, pain relief remained limited for most people, especially infants and children. Many denominations of the Christian Church viewed medical advances with skepticism. Even use of anesthesia during surgery was controversial.

PAIN IN THE EARLY 19ᵀᴴ CENTURY

Two earlier, albeit somewhat contradictory, views about pain continued in the 19th century. One view considered that pain was a punishment, which could be inflicted by God upon an individual who had sinned or more generally upon all of mankind, due to man's inherent sinfulness after the fall of Adam and Eve. (1)

The other view was that pain was a blessing, bestowed by God to bring people closer to Christ. John Henry Newman (1801-1890) was an influential Anglican priest who converted to Catholicism late in life and subsequently became a Cardinal in the Catholic Church. He preached, as many clerics had done for centuries, that "affliction is sent for our own personal good." (2) Newman wrote, as St. Paul had said, "If we suffer, we shall also reign with Him." (3) In other words, pain could be a blessing and have a positive effect. But Newman also wrote that pain "has no sanctifying influence in itself. Bad men are made worse by it....Nay, I would go so far as to say, not only that pain does not commonly improve us, but that without care it has a strong tendency to do our souls harms, viz., by making us selfish; an effect produced, even when it does us good in other ways." (4) Newman preached that in Christians, "Pain is no longer a curse, a necessary evil to be undergone with a dry submission or passive endurance – it may be considered even as a blessing of the Gospel." He also wrote that "the Gospel...has aided especially our view of the *sufferings* to which human nature is subjected; turning a punishment into a privilege, in the case of all pain, and especially of bodily pain." (4)

The idea that pain could be blessing expanded in the 19th century to encompass the view that God inflicted severe pain only in the elected few, i.e., whose who had been selected as "worthy of emulating the divine model." (5) A common theme in literature at this time centered on the pious invalid, who suffered nobly from unrelieved pain. This invalid, often a woman, was viewed as the modern "epitome of Christian sainthood." (6)

However, more secular ideas about pain started to gain strength in the 19th century, accompanying the newer view that the ability of humans to reason was a gift from God. Many people now felt that this gift of reason should be used to increase scientific and medical knowledge in order to reduce human pain and suffering.

DISCOVERY OF ANESTHESIA
IN THE MID-19ᵀᴴ CENTURY

The remarkable discovery of anesthesia in the 19ᵗʰ century was one of the greatest all-time scientific advancements in the history of pain and in the overall history of medicine. It was dentists who performed the first experiments with both nitrous oxide (laughing gas) and ether to try to reduce pain.

In 1844, Horace Wells, a dentist in Hartford, CT, observed that a young man who was under the influence of inhaled nitrous oxide did not appear to feel pain from a severe leg injury. Based on this observation, Wells directed his colleague Dr. Garner Colton to administer nitrous oxide to him when he had a wisdom tooth extracted. Since he had felt no pain, Wells did not believe the tooth had actually been removed until he saw the tooth himself! Dr. Colton went on to successfully use nitrous oxide to reduce dental pain in many of his patients. Unfortunately, when Dr. Wells attempted to demonstrate the utility of nitrous oxide for preventing pain in a patient at the Massachusetts General Hospital in Boston, his experiment failed, and nitrous oxide temporarily fell out of favor. (7)

Shortly thereafter, the dentist William Morton successfully demonstrated in 1846 that another inhaled substance (ether) could reduce dental pain. Morton subsequently served as an anesthetist, delivering ether during a variety of surgeries in Boston. Many patients proclaimed that they had felt no pain during these procedures! (7) Interestingly, the first modern use of the word "anesthesia" was in a letter written by the physician, poet, and professor Oliver Wendell Holmes to Dr. Morton in 1846. Holmes developed this term, based on the Greek word meaning "lack of sensation." (8)

News of the effectiveness of ether to reduce pain during surgery spread rapidly in both the United States and Britain. Only two months after Morton's demonstration in Boston that ether reduced pain during a variety of dental and surgical procedures, the London surgeon Robert Liston successfully utilized ether to eliminate pain during a leg amputation. (9)

Unfortunately, use of ether at this time was not always effective or without problems. Physicians, surgeons, and dentists did not understand how ether was working or know the best way to use it. In 1847, chloroform also began to be used as an anesthetic, but lack of understanding and imprecise methods resulted in some deaths. (10) The best methods to achieve effective anesthesia had not yet been developed.

Despite problems due to unoptimized methods, patients began to demand anesthetics, as news of the ability to reduce pain during surgery continued to spread. Now physicians and surgeons could eliminate pain during surgery. They had the tremendous power to decide which patients would suffer and who would not. (11) Certainly, a variety of criteria were used to determine which patients would benefit from the use of anesthesia. As Martin Pernick wrote in his book entitled *The Calculus of Suffering*, "Anesthesia won acceptance with a speed unprecedented in the history of pre-20th century medical innovation. Yet surgeons used it conservatively and selectively." (12) Indeed, leading hospitals in the United States did not rapidly adopt the universal use of anesthesia during surgery. Almost 1/3 of patients undergoing major surgery, especially amputations, at New York Hospital from 1847-1852, Massachusetts General Hospital in 1847, and Pennsylvania Hospital from 1853-1862 did not receive anesthesia. (13) At the extreme, perhaps surgeons may have even used anesthesia to reward a cooperative patient or withhold it to punish an uncooperative patient.

In the 19th century, chloroform began to be used to control the pain of childbirth. But most doctors were reluctant to use chloroform during childbirth, maintaining that labor pains were natural and should simply be endured. The most famous advocate was the British Queen Victoria. (10, 14) Although she was strongly advised against it on both medical and theological grounds, Queen Victoria requested and received chloroform for the birth of some of her children. (10, 14) She spoke in glowing terms about the value of chloroform to ease the pain of childbirth. (14)

Many people at this time believed that all pain was natural, not just the pain of childbirth. The idea that pain was an essential part of life and normal physiology may have contributed to the aversion to anesthesia. Both physicians and patients were often reluctant to utilize anesthesia during surgery. Some patients associated lack of pain sensation with impending death, since people near death often lose all sensations. In contrast, pain was viewed as a sign of life, predicting prompt healing and recovery. As a result, many people in the 19th century felt that anesthesia could hinder healing by abolishing the pain considered to be essential for complete recovery. (15)

Nevertheless, the discovery of anesthesia not only enabled pain-free surgery but also increased medical understanding of diseases. Before anesthesia, many physicians believed that diseases were simply a combination of physical symptoms such as pain. (12) The observation that pain could be eliminated without affecting the disease itself was surprising at this time. (12)

CONFLICT BETWEEN RELIGION AND ADVANCES IN MEDICINE IN THE 19TH CENTURY

By the latter half of the 19th century, much of the general population actively sought pain relief using the medical advances of the era. Most physicians and many theologians supported use of the newly discovered ways to reduce illness and pain. However, the ability to alleviate pain also renewed the conflict with the Christian belief that physical suffering could be linked to spiritual holiness, as discussed earlier in the chapter. (10, 15, 16)

This religious view played a role in the slow adoption of anesthesia. William Henry Atkinson, who became the first president of the American Dental Association in 1860, stated: "I think anesthesia is of the devil....I wish there were no such thing as anesthesia! I do not think men should be prevented from passing through what God intended them to endure." (17) Many other people also rejected the use of anesthesia, based on the continued belief that pain was God-given and brought people closer to God. Patrick McGrath and Anita Unruh wrote in a chapter on the history of pain that "to seek relief of pain often floundered on the boundary between necessary medical assistance and the perceived interference with the will of God." (18)

Hospitals established by the Catholic Church were filled with religious symbols to encourage the sick and dying to ponder the status of their souls. The Catholic Church in 19th-century France considered that the primary role of a physician caring for the dying was to maintain the patient's clarity of mind until his confession could be heard. It was important that the dying patient sought forgiveness of sins and received the last rites in a conscious state. (19) The Benedictine Peter Flood stated pain relief should never be provided to a sinner who had not confessed his sins. He wrote that a "man's eternal salvation" is "of more importance than any temporal ease." (20) However, if the patient's pain reduced his ability to give a clear confession, then the physician could provide pain-relieving medications, but only limited amounts that did not impair the patient's thinking. (19)

Throughout the centuries, Catholic nuns were often nurses. "Nursing nuns," along with the physicians, were expected to ensure that dying Catholics were able to receive the last rites as well as to convert non-religious patients to Catholicism. (21) During the Middle Ages and into the modern era, nuns held the keys to the dispensary, so they had tremendous power in utilizing the available medicinal extracts to relieve pain. They could selectively utilize these medicines at their discretion. (21)

Some patients, who perceived that they were dying, rejected pain-relieving agents due to concern that they would hinder their ability to fully experience the transition from life on earth to eternal life. Thomas "Stonewall" Jackson, a Confederate general in the American Civil War, reportedly refused chloroform when his arm was to be amputated because he did not want to "enter eternity in such a condition." (22) Similarly, the 19th-century Protestant Mary Rankin, who believed in the power of suffering to enhance spirituality, wrote in her autobiography that she refused even wine to blunt the pain of an upcoming amputation. She wrote: "I did not wish to be lulled to sleep; for if I died during the operation, I wished to have my senses about me at the time, and not pass into the world of spirits in a state of unconsciousness." (23)

EMERGENCE OF "FAITH CURE" AND THE CHRISTIAN SCIENCE CHURCH

In the late 19th century, a new movement began among evangelical Protestant Churches in the United States, and then spread to Great Britain and continental Europe. This movement taught that complete commitment to the teachings of Jesus Christ could bring relief from suffering and cure illness. Modern medical methods were not needed, since God as the "Great Physician" would heal the sick. This belief was often called "divine healing" or "faith cure." (24)

This rejection of modern medicine was not the same as the earlier Christian concepts that suffering should be simply endured, because either it could lead to holiness or it was a punishment. Rather, as the historian Heather Curtis wrote, a central tenet of this movement was "that protracted suffering was not God's will for anyone and therefore it must be God's will to heal." (25) Moreover, this new religion held "a model of spiritual experience that entailed active service to God rather than passive acceptance of pain." (26) Proponents of this new religion provided numerous examples of its

success in restoring health to those who previously had been seriously incapacitated and had suffered from severe pain. (24)

However, the prayers of those who believed in "faith cure" did
not always lead to healing. As a result, some individuals felt that
they had been abandoned by "the Great Physician." Others felt
that the failure of the faith cure must be their own fault! (27) Such
self-doubt and self-blame likely caused further suffering for those
who were not cured. As Curtis wrote: "It seems fair to suggest that
faith cure helped foster disparaging attitudes toward the body in
pain that have persisted throughout the twentieth and twenty-first
centuries." (27) I would argue that this was especially true for individuals who suffer from severe pain not attributable to an obvious
physical cause and for those suffering from mental illness.

I suggest that the faith cure movement caused more suffering
than purported healing. An example is my own mother, who suffered from episodes of severe depression throughout her life. She
was exposed to the faith cure movement in the 20th century by a
well-meaning friend. My mom was a devout Christian who diligent-
ly prayed for healing, but it didn't come. Through the remainder of
her life, she continued to blame herself for the recurrent episodes
of depression, in turn causing even more suffering.

The Christian Science movement was founded in 1879. It was
similar, but distinct from faith cure. In fact, proponents of faith
cure and Christian Science had a contentious relationship, with dis-
putes over fine points of doctrine. (24) The founder of the Christian
Science religion, Mary Baker Eddy, had a strict Calvinist upbringing
in the Congregational Church and studied the Bible from an early
age. As a child, she believed in a "merciless" God. (28) As an adult,
she moved from her earlier belief that suffering was God's will,
towards the belief that it was God's will to be healed from sickness and infirmities. As in the faith cure movement, the Christian
Science religion believed that modern medicine was not needed to

treat diseases and relieve suffering. Instead, healing would come from prayer and studying the Bible, especially the teachings of Jesus Christ. (24, 29)

The headquarters of the Christian Science Church are in Boston, but branches are found throughout the world. Mary Baker Eddy's seminal work, entitled *Science and Health,* was originally published in 1875 under her name from her first marriage. (29) This book has since been published in seventeen languages and continues to inspire members of this religion. Later editions include testimonies by members of the Christian Science Church which state that their study of *Science and Health* has enhanced their relationship with God, resulting in healing of various types of diseases, both physical and mental. (30)

CONFLICT BETWEEN RELIGIOUS VIEWS AND PAIN RELIEF IN THE EARLY 20TH CENTURY

The belief that illness, pain, and suffering could be relieved through faith alone continued within the Christian Science Church. Confronting the emergence of "faith healing," some eminent British physicians wrote that "faith," in the broader sense, could play a role in the practice of medicine. For example, faith that a patient has in his physician can contribute to healing. (31) Another prominent physician pointed out that the concept of "faith healing" is not new or limited to the Christian Science Church, since healing through faith (via rituals) has existed along with the practice of medicine throughout the history of the Western world. (32)

Other physicians in the early 20th century continued to believe that pain served a noble purpose. One such physician was John M.T. Finney. He was professor of clinical surgery at the Johns Hopkins Hospital in the US and also a renowned Presbyterian churchman. He delivered the prestigious 1914 Ether Day Lecture at the Massachusetts General Hospital. Although in his lecture he did acknowledge the considerable benefit of pain relief, he also believed that pain has value, stating that pain has a "refining and ennobling" influence. (33, 34) Decades later, the *British Medical Journal* published a letter to the editor by the physician Paul C. Gibson entitled "Divine Healing." In this 1956 letter, Dr. Gibson stated: "If we know, as we should do if we have studied humanity carefully and intelligently, that lasting joy only comes through pain, we should not ask for relief from pain but rather for grace to endure it." (35)

Some Protestant clergy in the early 20th century continued to preach that pain was a gift from God. The noted Christian thinker and author C.S. Lewis published a philosophical and theological book in 1944 entitled *The Problem of Pain*. (36) This book pondered the age-old question: Why should an omnipotent and benevolent God allow people to suffer? The author concluded that human pain must be serving a higher purpose, which we do not fully understand.

The Catholic Church also continued to teach that pain and suffering can have a divine purpose. In a textbook written in 1949 primarily for Catholic nurses, the author wrote "the true follower of Christ sees in suffering a stepping-stone to holiness, a divine invitation to spiritual greatness." (37) He went on to write that the Catholic nurse *will* do everything she can to relieve pain, but when this is not achieved, she will provide comfort to the patients by reminding them that "they may use pain as means of spiritual union with God." (37)

A book written in 1960 as part of a series entitled *The 20th Century Encyclopedia of Catholicism* stated: "From the theological aspect, it seems that pain has a wider purpose and function. It is man's lot to suffer." The author continued: "It is the proper talk of the doctor to relieve pain....How does the doctor's talk of relieving pain equate with the patient's duty to accept suffering? There is in reality no conflict here....But has the patient the obligation to accept this relief? Not so, for he may choose to bear the suffering in expiation of his sins, to gain merit for himself, and to fulfill the divine command to shoulder his cross." Necessary acceptance of suffering is an integral part of the Christian life. (38) This author went on to say that individuals may "fulfil this obligation to bear the cross in many other ways," besides accepting suffering from pain. (38) Nevertheless, such teaching from the Church likely caused concern among devout Catholics about the use of anesthesia or pain-relieving medications.

Apparently, such concerns led Pope Pius XII to write the following in 1960: "The patient, desirous of avoiding or of relieving pain, may, without any disquietude of conscience, use the means discovered by science which in themselves are not immoral." (38) It is amazing that even in the mid-20th century some people needed such reassurance from a high religious authority that it was acceptable to utilize modern pain-relieving methods.

Late in the 20th century, the Catholic Church continued to state that pain and suffering can be a blessing. In 1990, Pope John Paul II wrote: "What we express with the word pain is essential to the nature of Man. Sharing in the sufferings of Christ is also suffering for the Kingdom of God. In the just eyes of God...those who share in Christ's sufferings become worthy of this Kingdom. Through their pain they pay back the boundless price of our redemption. Pain is an appeal to Man's moral greatness and spiritual maturity." (39)

LIMITED PAIN CONTROL IN INFANTS AND CHILDREN IN THE 19TH AND 20TH CENTURIES

Most people today would be astonished and horrified to learn that until very recently, little or no consideration was given to infants' pain. The standard of care for infants and children in the late 19th and much of the 20th centuries often did not include analgesia or even anesthesia for some painful procedures, including surgeries.

A disturbing example is a chapter written by WE Casselberry in a pediatric textbook published in 1898. (40) This chapter discussed various procedures for tonsillectomies, which were common surgeries at this time. Casselberry wrote: "an anesthetic is not usually necessary when the faucial tonsils alone are to be abscised." He went on to describe specific instruments to be used and wrote "The tonsillotome is still the best implement for children who are not anesthetized, because of the rapidity, precision, and comparative ease with which this method can be practiced....The pain is not really great." (40) How in the world did Dr. Casselberry know that the pain experienced by the un-anesthetized child was not great?

Somewhat later, Dr. Max Thorek wrote in a book entitled *Modern Surgical Technique* that "often no anesthetic is required" when operating on young infants: indeed "a sucker consisting of a sponge dipped in some sugar water will often suffice to calm the baby." (41-43)

Post-surgical pain in children also received little attention. As recently as 1968, only 3% of children received pain-relieving medications after various surgical procedures. (44) Even after major surgery, many children did not receive any analgesic medications. Over half of the children (ages 4-8) in a 1977 study received no medications for post-operative pain. (45) Moreover, most of the children who had been given physicians' orders for analgesics did not actually receive the prescribed medications while in the hospital. (45) The authors of this study concluded that it appears "nursing personnel were reluctant to exercise their prerogative to give medication," as prescribed by the physicians. Interestingly, the same study found that adults with the same diagnoses received an average of thirty-seven doses of pain-relieving medications per person compared with an average of less than one dose per child. This was in spite of the fact that the adults and children were being cared for by the same nursing and medical staff in the same hospital. (45)

Clearly, children were not receiving appropriate pain care. Another study at this time found that 12% of children who had open heart surgery were not given any post-surgical analgesics. (46)

Apparently, these were not isolated examples. A 1994 article in the *New England Journal of Medicine* stated: "There are large discrepancies between the amounts of postoperative analgesia ordered for and administered to adults and those ordered for and administered to children who have the same diagnoses and have undergone the same procedures." (47)

Why Wasn't Pain Control Considered Important for Infants?

Pain control for infants was particularly lacking. Many reasons were given by the medical community for the lack of concern about infants' pain. Among these were that it is difficult to measure pain in infants and that drugs to relieve pain are too dangerous for sick babies. Other reasons given were: when a baby cries, it does not necessarily mean that he is in pain since babies also cry under other situations; pediatric physicians and nurses would not be able to handle their emotions if they thought that the infants indeed did feel pain; medical personnel are too busy "saving lives," especially in neonatal intensive care units, to pay attention to possible pain. (48)

But the main reason for the apparently callous disregard for infants' pain was that medical personnel believed that young infants were essentially unable to feel pain. Pediatric medicine in the mid-20th century taught that young infants did not have fully developed nervous systems and therefore could not truly experience pain. (48-50) The view was that even though it might appear that an infant was in pain, the behaviors were only primitive reflexes, not really indicative of pain. (48-50) In a 1986 study, 40% of family practitioners, surgeons and pediatricians believed that newborns did not experience pain in the first month of life. (51) As a result, standard medical practice in the 1980s provided only minimal anesthesia to newborns undergoing surgery and essentially no pain management after the operation. (50)

Pediatric textbooks in the middle of the 20th century mentioned pain in only a few places and then only to aid in the diagnosis of a particular disease. (45, 50, 52, 53) Out of a total of 12,000 pages in ten leading pediatric textbooks in use in 1987, only a single page dealt with pain relief! (54)

Beginning of Changing Attitudes and Medical Practice for Pain Relief in Infants

However, by the late 1980s, some in the medical community began to believe that infants could feel real pain and therefore should receive anesthesia and/or analgesia. Between 1985 and 1988, leading medical journals published editorials and commentaries calling attention to the issue of pain in infants. One of these commentaries in the journal *Pediatrics* stated that although many hospitalized infants did experience severe pain, most did not receive appropriate and adequate medications for pain relief. (54) The commentary said: "This maltreatment reaches cruel proportions in infants and neonates when surgical procedures are sometime performed without anesthesia and postoperative analgesia." (54)

Although the medical community in the late 1980s was beginning to pay more attention to the pain of infants, it was really the activism of a woman named Jill Lawson that led to major changes both in public awareness and medical practice. Ms. Lawson was the mother of a premature infant who underwent numerous surgical procedures. After the baby's death, Lawson requested and reviewed the medical history. To her astonishment and horror, the medical records revealed that the infant had not received any anesthesia during the multiple surgeries! After the *Washington Post* published her story in 1986 (55), there was considerable public outrage. (56) Lawson continued to advocate for pain control for infants through letters to editors of major medical journals such as *Lancet* (57) and *The New England Journal of Medicine*. (58) Accordingly, through her activism, Lawson played a major role in changing the practice of medicine for neonates. (56)

Scientific and medical understanding of pediatric pain increased substantially at the end of the 20th century. One of the earliest studies, which demonstrated that the physiological effects of painful medical procedures in newborns were similar to those in adults, was published in 1989. (59) Today, we know that the nervous systems of preterm and full-term infants are sufficiently developed so that infants can feel pain. (60) Current understanding is that pain pathways are active and functional in neonates at the cortical level and are not simply reflexes, even as early as twenty-five weeks' gestation. (61)

Clinical studies in the 1980s demonstrated that adequate pain prevention for infants during surgery resulted in better overall medical outcomes. (62, 63) For example, adding a pain-relieving medicine (the opioid fentanyl) to the standard minimal anesthesia was advantageous for premature babies. (63) However, this study caused wide outcry from the public and the press. (63) So, in spite of increased knowledge and advocacy, it was still highly controversial in the late 20th century to provide effective pain relief to young babies.

Long-Term Effects of Pain in Infants and Children

In addition to the immediate suffering, inadequate pain control can have long-lasting negative effects on infants and children, since their nervous systems are still developing. The multiple painful procedures which premature or seriously ill infants undergo may cause permanent structural and functional changes. (64) A recent policy statement by the American Academy of Pediatrics emphasized not only that ethical considerations call for pain prevention in neonates, but also that unrelieved pain can alter nervous system development and cause later abnormal responses to stress, which can persist long into childhood. (65)

For example, two interesting studies demonstrated the negative consequences of painful procedures in infants. In one study, newborns, who underwent repeated heel lancing for blood collection in the first 24 to 36 hours of life, exhibited greater pain responses during subsequent venipunctures than infants who had not undergone early painful procedures. (66) In the other study, circumcised babies cried longer and showed more signs of discomfort 4-6 months later during routine vaccinations than non-circumcised infants. (67) But babies who had an anesthetic cream applied locally prior to circumcision showed less discomfort during the later vaccinations, demonstrating that it was the pain during circumcision, not the procedure itself, which caused much of the distress during the later painful procedures. (67) Research studies such as these led to increased attention to pain control in infants.

GENDER BIAS IN PAIN RELIEF?

Relief of pain during childbirth continued to be controversial in the early 20th century. In 1934, Dame Louise McIlroy wrote in the Forward to the textbook *Anaesthesia and Analgesia in Labour*, "No painful operation nowadays is contemplated without the aid of sedatives and anesthetics. Why, therefore, in these days of enlightenment has so little consideration been given to child birth with regards to measures of relief?" (68) Was it because of historic religious views, concerns that anesthesia during childbirth might be harmful to the child, or was there gender bias in not providing pain relief to the mother?

Some physicians exhibited a moralistic and patronizing attitude toward women and were reluctant to provide them with pain-relieving medications. In 1904, the well-known physician Silas Weir

Mitchell published a book for the lay public entitled *Doctor and Patient*. (69) The focus of the book was that women need to endure pain themselves and then ensure that their children receive proper upbringing so that they could also endure pain. He stated in his book: "Even if it [pain] recur at intervals... in the name of reason let him ['the wise physician'] be the sole judge of your need to be relieved by drugs. He well knows, as you cannot know, that the frequent use of morphia [morphine] seems in the end to increase, not to lessen, the whole amount of probably future pain, and that which eases for a time is a devil in angelic disguise." (70) Of course, this paternalistic statement could be based on concerns about the dangers of morphine, but nevertheless this book is directed solely to women.

As discussed in Chapter 5, fibromyalgia (FM) is a major type of chronic pain affecting ~7 times more women than men. Since usually there is no readily identifiable cause, FM has been broadly misunderstood and often considered to be purely psychosomatic. Perhaps gender bias has contributed to the frequent dismissal of this type of pain that does not have actual physical manifestations.

A more complete discussion about gender bias in pain management is beyond the scope of this book.

RISE IN USE OF OPIOIDS FOR PAIN RELIEF

The extract from poppies, known as opium, was used since antiquity to relieve pain, diarrhea, and various nervous conditions. Opium became one of the most important medications in the 19th and early 20th centuries. In an article published in 1915 in the prestigious *Journal of the American Medical Association*, a physician wrote as follows: "If the entire *materia medica* at our disposal were limited to the choice and use of only one drug, I am sure that a great many, if not the majority, of us would choose opium." (71)

In the early 19th century, morphine (the active ingredient in opium) was isolated and began to be used as a pure medicinal compound for a variety of disorders. Subsequently, use of morphine increased rapidly in both Europe and the United states. Morphine was the major ingredient in widely available medicines such as Mrs. Winslow's Soothing Syrup and Kopp's Baby Friend. (72) Physicians routinely and readily provided morphine, especially to middle-aged middle-class women, in the mid-late 19th century for a variety of physical and psychological pains. (73) In general, there was little concern about the negative aspects of morphine at this time, although certainly they were known. But we must remember that there were few alternatives to morphine for pain relief even towards the end of the 19th century. Aspirin did not become available until the late 1890s and acetaminophen was not commercialized until the mid-20th century.

In England, something known as the Brompton cocktail, which was composed of morphine, cocaine, cannabis, gin, syrup and chloroform, became widely used in the early 20th century to alleviate pain in the dying. Clifford Hoyle from the Brompton Hospital, which gave its name to the cocktail, stated repeatedly that pain-relieving agents, whether wine, whiskey, opioids or others, should be freely provided to the dying. (74) By 1935, St. Luke's Hospital in London was actively using the Brompton cocktail. (75) Later studies demonstrated that the Brompton cocktail was not more effective than morphine alone, and the cocktail fell from favor. Nevertheless, use of the Brompton cocktail continued at some British clinics and hospitals into the 1980s. (75)

As use of morphine expanded, problems of abuse became more widely known. Eventually in 1970, the United States adopted the Controlled Substances Act to reduce illicit trafficking of opioids and other drugs with abuse potential. Current issues and controversies associated with use of opioids for pain relief are discussed extensively in Chapter 7.

PAIN RELIEF IN THE LATTER PART
OF THE 20ᵀᴴ CENTURY

Substantial strides were made in the latter part of the 20th century in recognizing the importance of pain and pain relief. Three women, Margo McCaffery, R.N., Dame Cicely Saunders, M.D., and Anne Merriman, M.D. were especially notable in bringing the problem of pain to the attention of the public.

"Pain Is What the Patient Says It Is"

Margo McCaffery was a pioneer in pain management nursing in the US. She developed a definition which had a major impact on prevailing attitudes toward pain and pain management. In 1968 she stated: "Pain is whatever the experiencing person says it is and exists whenever he says it does." (76) This was an important statement, since there was no objective way to measure pain in 1968. Unfortunately, this is still true today. As a result, clinicians still have to rely on the patient's self-report and assume that it is true. But, as discussed in Chapter 5, physicians often doubt patients' own statements about their pain. Nevertheless, McCaffery's definition of pain helped provide legitimacy to patients' self-reported pain.

In her seminal book, McCaffery stated that the patient must always be believed, even if no cause could be identified for the pain. She made an important analogy to the modern judicial system, in which a person is considered innocent until proven guilty. Similarly, her definition of pain means that "the patient's report of pain is never doubted – the patient is always believed." (76) She acknowledged that this could result in believing lies expressed by malingerers, who falsely claim to be in pain for dishonest purposes such as attempts to obtain disability status or to receive drugs. However, she goes on to state that there are very few such malingerers. So even if a few people do exploit false claims about pain, this is a small risk compared with the large number of people truly in pain who will receive the care and concern they deserve. (76)

By the end of the 20th century, pain relief had become a high priority in the United States. In 1996, the American Pain Society designated pain as "the fifth vital sign." This designation meant that a health care provider should ask a patient about his pain when evaluating the other vital signs; i.e., pulse rate, respiration rate, temperature and blood pressure. Calling pain a vital sign acknowledged the importance of pain in a person's overall health and well-being. This new emphasis on pain and pain relief was certainly a shift from earlier times. However, as discussed in Chapter 5, this view appears to have been short-lived, due primarily to the rise in opioid abuse.

Birth of the Hospice Movement and Palliative Care

The pioneering work of Dame Cicely Saunders, MD and her colleagues led to the world's first modern hospice, St. Christopher's, which opened in London in 1967, to reduce pain for the terminally ill. The term *hospice* comes from the Latin and Greek words meaning hospitality. As such, the hospice movement is based on the relationship between the caregiver (the host) and the patient (the guest) to provide holistic care for all the needs of the patient. (77)

Dr. Saunders has been called "the first modern doctor to dedicate her entire career to caring for those at the end of life." (78) Following the example of St. Christopher's, the hospice movement has become widespread throughout the Western world. St. Christopher's has also served as a training ground for many of the health care providers who developed the related medical discipline known as palliative care. The term *palliative* comes from the Latin word *pall,* meaning blanket. Palliative care means providing comfort to those suffering, such as the comfort provided by a blanket. (77)

Both the hospice movement and palliative care expanded in the Western world in the 1970s and 1980s, especially for patients with advanced cancer. But in much of the world, dying patients still suffered from excruciating pain. Anne Merriman, a British doctor who specialized in providing pain relief for the dying, recognized that dying cancer patients in Africa had little or no pain relief. In addition, the AIDS epidemic was raging in Africa, with most patients dying in extreme pain. In 1993, Merriman founded Hospice Africa in Uganda. (79)

In spite of seemingly unsurmountable difficulties, Dr. Merriman established hospice and palliative care not only in Uganda, but also in other African countries and some Asian countries. Through sheer determination, she enabled many dying patients to obtain relief from pain and suffering. (77, 79) She had to deal with fear of opioids, since aversion to opioids was pervasive in Africa. She also developed a simple, inexpensive method for delivering morphine in a liquid form for patients to drink. Different strengths of morphine were coded via different food colorings, which made them easy to identify by hospice workers and patients, reducing mix-ups. This method is still in use today. (79)

In contrast with opioid abuse in many developed countries today, Merriman stated that there were no diversions or addictions among the 24,000 hospice patients who had been prescribed morphine. (79) Instead, she said that in 2016 the biggest problem in Africa was the limited number of doctors available to care for the many patients needing palliative care. (79)

CONCLUSION

As discussed in this chapter and the preceding one, many views have existed about pain and pain relief through the centuries. For more than 2000 years, many philosophers and theologians in the Western World have debated the meaning of pain, even whether pain should be alleviated. For centuries, the Christian Church assigned a higher purpose to pain. Teaching that pain was a blessing or a punishment may have had the intended effect; i.e., leading people to live more moral lives. However, it is likely that viewing pain as God-given also caused unnecessary suffering, through reluctance to use pain-relieving methods.

The discovery of anesthesia in the 19th century was a major milestone in medicine. The effect of this discovery on prevention of pain during surgery is unequaled. It seems unimaginable today that in earlier times surgeries were performed on patients who were conscious!

In actual practice, pain prevention and relief continued to be controversial and uneven in the 19th and much of the 20th centuries. In particular, pain relief in infants and children was limited. It was not until that the latter half of the 20th century that the importance of pain relief for everyone became widely accepted by both physicians and the public.

CHAPTER 4

PAIN IN ANIMALS

Human pain is the focus of this book, but what about pain in other creatures? The present chapter briefly describes that very little attention has been paid to animal pain in the past, even as recently as the mid-20th century. This is in part because animals may not express pain in the same way as humans. For example, animals may instinctively hide their pain to reduce their vulnerability to attack by enemies. It is certainly common for even domestic animals to not vocalize when they are in pain and instead to simply retreat to a quiet place alone. But there are other reasons that pain in animals has been neglected and under-treated.

HISTORICAL VIEWS REGARDING ANIMAL PAIN

As discussed in earlier chapters, Christianity often taught that human pain can serve a moral or divine purpose. This was difficult to reconcile with pain in animals. In the 17th and 18th centuries, there were heated philosophical debates about whether non-human animals actually do experience pain. Since animals were not considered to have souls or free will to choose between good and evil, why should God allow them to suffer? (1) This was still a subject of debate in the 20th century. C.S. Lewis wrote in 1944 that "so far as we know beasts are incapable either of sin or virtue: therefore they can neither deserve pain nor be improved by it." (2) He further argued that although painful conditions might exist, the animals do not actually "feel pain" because they do not integrate sensations into their consciousness. (2)

Of course, when our pets simply retreat from sight or cry and moan after an injury, we assume that indeed they are in pain. But is this pain somehow different from human pain? It was once thought that the responses of animals to injury were simply reflexes and did not mean that the animals were actually in pain. However, we now know that the systems which transmit nerve impulses from the site of injury to specific regions in the brain, generating the sensation of pain, are basically the same in humans and many other animals. (3, 4) But, as discussed in Chapter 1, pain is complex and human emotions can strongly affect pain sensation. Although we cannot really understand emotions in other creatures and how animal emotions impact their pain, it is clear that humans and many other animals have the same basic physiological mechanisms which generate pain.

SURGICAL AND POST-SURGICAL PAIN IN ANIMALS IN THE 20TH CENTURY

In the early 20th century, there was little concern about the pain of animals, even those undergoing surgical procedures. Although general anesthesia was almost universally used by this time for major human surgery, anesthesia was not widely adopted by the veterinary profession until much later.

A series of veterinary books published between 1900 and 1910 described many surgical interventions for a variety of common ailments affecting domestic animals. For example, the earliest publications in the series described in detail multiple types of surgeries on the legs of horses to correct injuries, congenital malformations, or infections, but there was no mention of pain prevention or pain relief. (5) The emphasis was on enabling the horses to get back to work, with no apparent concern about the pain accompanying the surgeries!

A 1906 textbook emphasized the importance of animal restraint during surgery. The primary purpose of restraint was to control the animal so that the veterinarian could perform surgery without harm to *himself*. (6) Anesthesia was briefly mentioned, but the author wrote: "In veterinary surgery, the indication for anesthesia, has not, to the same extent as in human, the avoidance of pain in the patient for its object, and though the duties of the veterinarian include that of avoiding the infliction of *unnecessary* pain as much as possible, the administration of anesthetic compounds aims principally to facilitate the performance of the operation for its own sake, by depriving the patient of the power of obstructing, and perhaps even frustrating its execution, to his own detriment, by the violence of his struggles, and the persistency of his resistance." (6) The main concerns were a successful operation and the safety of the veterinarian; the suffering of the animal was of little consequence.

Castration is a common surgery for companion animals and some farm animals, but anesthesia for this type of surgery was particularly slow to be adopted. A veterinary textbook published early in the 20th century stated that anesthesia is not used for castration of dogs unless "there exists some pathological condition which renders the operation painful and tedious." (7) Similarly, this author wrote that "No anesthesia is necessary for castration of the cat under normal conditions." (7)

Finally, by the middle of the 20th century, textbooks did acknowledge pain in animals and recommended the use of local anesthetics for minor surgical procedures and general anesthesia for
all but the simplest procedures. A veterinary textbook published in
1953 stated: "Anesthesia for operations on animals is....as essential
to control pain in animals during an operation as it is in humans."
(8) Nevertheless, the actual practice often lagged behind textbook
guidance. Authors of a chapter in a recent textbook stated that "It
is sad to say, but a 'heavy hand', without analgesia/anesthesia or
even sedation, was the stock in trade of many 'large animal' prac-
ticing veterinarians well into the latter half of the 20th century." (9)
The authors went on to say that "the modern era of veterinary anesthesia was [only] initiated during the last three decades of the
20th century." (9)

In a memoir published by a veterinary surgeon in 1952, he described his early experience in castrating horses and cows using a
knife and a red-hot iron, with no anesthesia. (10) He wrote "the accepted axiom in my youth was that pain was regrettable but necessary" in castration of farm animals. (10) Pain was minimized only by
the speed of the veterinarian performing the surgery!

Some types of surgeries on farm animals are often performed by
farmers themselves. This is especially true for castrations. Practical
guides published in the mid-20th century for farmers contained detailed information on castration methodology for a variety of young
farm animals but did not describe use of anesthesia or other pain-
relieving methods. (11-14) One of the books stated, "the whole job
takes only seconds for the experienced person" to perform (14),
implying that there was no need to be concerned about pain the
animal might be experiencing. My brothers and cousins who routinely performed hog castrations on family farms in the 1960s and
1970s confirmed that indeed castrations were performed without
anesthesia. (15) Other commonly performed procedures such as

tail docking of lambs and dehorning of calves were also often performed by farmers without use of anesthesia. (11-14)

What about pain after surgery? Many veterinarians considered that post-operative pain "served a useful purpose by preventing activity that could cause further tissue injury." (16) So even though surgical anesthesia was becoming widely used by veterinarians in the mid- 20th century, medications to relieve pain after surgery were not routinely utilized.

Interestingly, the general anesthetic pentobarbital, which was commonly used in veterinary practice prior to the 1980s, produced prolonged sleep. As a result, some degree of post-operative pain relief probably existed due to the long-acting effect of this anesthetic. However, after the new shorter-acting anesthetics became more widely used, it is likely that animals experienced more post-operative pain as the effects of the anesthesia wore off.

Most dogs and cats undergoing surgery in a veterinary teaching hospital in the 1980s did not receive any pain-relieving medications after surgery. Only 29% of the dogs in this study received an analgesic after recovery from general anesthesia. (17) Even when medical records stated that the dogs *were* likely experiencing moderate to severe pain, only half received pain-relieving medications. It was even worse for cats; only one out of fifteen cats received an analgesic after surgery. (17)

MANAGEMENT OF PAINFUL DISEASES AND CONDITIONS IN ANIMALS IN THE 20TH CENTURY

In addition to surgical pain, many diseases and other conditions can cause severe pain in animals. The aforementioned series of veterinary surgical books published in the early 1900s noted that many of these conditions themselves could be painful, but there was very limited mention of medications to relieve pain. One exception was the recommendation that medications such as salicylate of soda, sulphate of quinine, antipyrine, and tincture of colchicum could be helpful in relieving pain associated with muscular rheumatism in horses and dogs. (18)

Even in the mid-20th century, non-surgical pain in animals received little attention. For example, there were no entries for analgesia or pain relief in the index of a 1953 textbook on veterinary medicine for dogs. (19) My scan of this book found that pain relief was mentioned for only two conditions. One was pleurisy, for which the authors stated that codeine or morphine can be used in "extreme cases" to relieve pain. (20) The other condition was enteritis, for which "tincture of camphorated opium" could be administered along with milk of bismuth and Kaopectate via a stomach tube, and if a "dog is uncooperative," morphine or Demoral could be administered prior to inserting the stomach tube. (21)

PAIN CONTROL IN ANIMALS IN THE 21ST CENTURY

Veterinarians and the public are now aware that other species besides humans do experience pain. As a result, pain prevention and relief for domestic animals have substantially improved over previous eras and continue to improve, although early in the 21st century, pain prevention and relief for animals were still woefully inadequate. A friend told me that after her dog was spayed in 2000, the veterinarian told her that he didn't think it would be painful and that no pain relief was needed after the surgery! (22) An article published in 2002 in the *Journal of the American Veterinary Association* said: "The current state of pain management in dogs and cats is uneven at best, ranging from the excellent use of pain control techniques by some veterinarians to the complete disregard of pain control by others." (23) The article also made the more general statement that in 2002 "it is estimated that few animals under veterinary care receive adequate pain control." (23)

Today, essentially all animal surgeries performed by veterinarians, including castration, are done under some type of anesthesia. This is both medically and ethically appropriate for the sake of the animals. Of course, anesthesia also enables veterinarians to perform complex technical procedures with greater accuracy.

Veterinarians' awareness of the importance of post-surgical pain control in animals has substantially increased in the 21st century. (23) A widely used veterinary textbook published in 2003 states that "it is now generally accepted that most animals benefit significantly if analgesia is routinely provided whenever pain is present," including after surgery. (16) A subsequent veterinary textbook published in 2015 concurs that pain relief should be provided to all animals after surgical procedures. (24) Both of these textbooks are solely devoted to anesthesia and analgesia in a variety of animal species, demonstrating that pain prevention and relief in animals are finally being taken seriously. (16, 24)

Veterinarians' knowledge and attitudes about pain improved between 2001 and 2012, especially for dogs and cats. (25) Today pain medications are usually provided to cats and dogs to relieve both post-operative pain and chronic pain resulting from cancer, arthritis, or other disorders. However, pain management for farm animals continues to be limited. Although the Farm Animal Welfare Council published the Five Freedoms of Farm Animals which included the "Freedom from Pain," the economics and profitability of farming are sometimes at odds with providing effective pain relief for farm animals. It is likely that there is a considerable disparity between providing adequate pain relief for companion animals versus farm animals. (26) For example, the customary relief provided to hogs for a variety of painful conditions is only anti-inflammatory medications (27), which, as in humans, will only relieve mild pain. If pain is more severe, euthanasia is often the practical option. (27)

CONCLUSION

Use of anesthesia and analgesia in animals lagged behind their use in humans and only became common at the end of the 20th century. Even in the 21st century, animals still may not receive adequate medications for pain relief. Nevertheless, the situation has substantially improved over previous eras and continues to improve.

As an animal lover, I conclude this chapter with a favorite quote from the naturalist Henry Beston about animals. "We patronize them for their incompleteness, for their tragic fate for having taken form so far below ourselves. And therein do we err....In a world older and more complete than ours, they move finished and complete, gifted with the extensions of the senses we have lost or never attained, living by voices we shall never hear. They are not brethren, they are not underlings: they are other nations, caught with ourselves in the net of life and time, fellow prisoners of the splendor and travail of the earth." (28) So we must treat our fellow creatures with respect and use our abilities as humans to treat them humanely, including relieving their pain and suffering as much as possible.

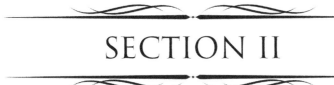

SECTION II

TREATMENT OF
PAIN TODAY

CHAPTER 5

PAIN AND PAIN RELIEF
IN THE 21ST CENTURY

Even with recent advances in nearly all areas of medicine, many people today continue to suffer from unrelieved pain. Pain is currently the most common health problem in the US and also one of the most expensive. Both acute pain and chronic pain are often inadequately relieved.

MANAGEMENT OF ACUTE PAIN IN HOSPITALS

Let's begin the discussion about the problem of unrelieved pain in the 21st century by evaluating pain management in hospitals. Most patients experience pain at least part of the time they are hospitalized. This pain can be the result of an accident, an acute painful condition, childbirth, pain following surgery and other causes. Certainly a hospital is not expected to be a "pain-free zone," but pain relief is often inadequate even in such a controlled clinical environment.

Unrelieved pain is a problem especially in emergency departments (ED) and intensive care units (ICU). A 1989 report from one
hospital found that over half of the patients complaining of pain did
not receive any analgesics while in the ED. (1) A 2007 study found
that more than 75% of patients in the ICU who had cardiac surgery
reported they had been in pain. (2) Disturbingly, the author of this
study wrote that there had been no substantial improvement in
pain control in the ICU since an earlier study in 1990. (2)

Inadequate pain management in hospitals is not limited to the
ED and ICU. A 2015 publication reported a 70% prevalence of pain
in hospitalized adult medical-surgical patients. (3) Nearly 50% of seriously ill adult patients in five teaching hospitals reported that they
were in pain, with almost 15% saying that they had extremely severe or moderately severe pain at least half the time. (4) An earlier
study found that more than half of such hospitalized patients described their pain as "excruciating" and that fewer than 50% were
even asked by a clinician whether they were in pain. (5)

Post-operative pain is often under-treated. A 2003 national
study found that approximately 80% of patients experienced pain
after surgery. (6) Although some level of pain is expected after surgery even if appropriate medications are provided, 86% of post-
surgical patients who experienced acute pain said that their pain
was moderate, severe, or even extreme. (6) Due to this woefully
inadequate pain relief, the American Pain Society, together with
the American Society of Anesthesiologists, published guidelines
for management of post-operative pain. (7) Hopefully these 2016
guidelines, which recommended a variety of pain-relieving methods, will become widely adopted and will lead to a reduction in
post-surgical pain.

The consequences of unrelieved post-operative pain go far
beyond the immediate distress. Inadequate pain relief can have
both physiologic and psychologic effects which delay recovery.

Unrelieved post-operative pain can also lead to development of chronic pain. (8) Indeed, 10-50% of patients who experience acute pain after common types of surgery go on to develop chronic pain. (9) Moreover, the greater the intensity of the acute pain, the more likely the patient will develop chronic pain. (9)

CANCER PAIN AND OTHER TYPES OF SEVERE PAIN

Pain is often the first symptom experienced by people with cancer, with increasing severity as the cancer progresses. According to an extensive review in 2007, over half of the cancer patients said that they were in pain, and more than 1/3 of these patients said the pain was moderate to severe. (10) An updated review of the prevalence of pain in cancer patients from 2007-2013 found that treatment of pain had improved, but still ~1/3 of the patients did not receive pain medications that were appropriate for the pain intensity. (11) Even when strong pain medications were provided to cancer patients in the last year of life, the medications were often given long after the onset of severe pain. (12)

Much of this suffering by cancer patients is avoidable. Experts have stated that adequate pain control could be achieved in 70-90% of cancer patients if guidelines by the World Health Organization were followed. (10, 13)

A survey of physicians in the Eastern Cooperative Oncology Group found that nearly all these cancer specialists felt that the majority of cancer patients were not receiving adequate pain medications. (14) Most of these physicians attributed the inadequate pain management to poor assessment of pain severity (14), likely due in part to the lack of methods which can accurately determine the severity. Other reasons cited were reluctance of patients to report their level of pain and to take pain-relieving medications, as well as reluctance of physicians to prescribe the strong opioids. (14)

In addition to cancer patients, many other people also experience severe pain. These include people with HIV/AIDS. Although antiretroviral drugs have extended the lives of those infected with HIV, many continue to live and die in pain. Up to 60-80% of AIDS patients with advanced disease suffer from intense pain. (15) In spite of pain management guidelines which call for the use of strong opioids to relieve severe pain, it has been reported that fewer than 8% of AIDS patients in severe pain actually received these medications. (16)

Injured soldiers returning from war often suffer from severe pain which can become chronic. According to a 2014 study, nearly half of the 2,500 US soldiers who recently returned from deployment in Afghanistan or Iraq had chronic pain. Many said they had pain daily or constantly, with 51% reporting that the pain was moderate or severe. (17)

As discussed in greater detail in the next two chapters, opioids effectively relieve severe pain. Although there are well-known risks associated with opioids, most health care providers consider that opioids are important drugs for relief of severe pain. Nevertheless, recent increased regulations and other factors are now limiting the availability of opioids for pain patients in the United States.

In most Western European countries, many types of opioids are readily available, especially for patients with cancer pain. (18) It is a different story in some Eastern European countries, with the Ukraine being the most restrictive. (18) The ability to obtain pain relief is even more dismal when one looks beyond Europe and the US. It is particularly alarming in the developing world. It has been estimated that 83% of the world's population lives in countries with little or no access to opioids. (19)

A study published in 2014 estimated the extent of adequate

pain relief in individual countries. This study compared the actual consumption of opioids in each country with the calculated needs, based on the prevalence of three major causes of moderate and severe pain: lethal injuries, terminal cancer, and end-stage HIV/AIDS. (20) There were extreme differences in opioid consumption. The US and Canada had extraordinarily high opioid consumption, whereas many European countries and Australia had what was considered approximately adequate consumption. Some other countries, especially Afghanistan, India, Senegal and Zambia, had less than 1% of the opioid consumption considered adequate for pain relief. (20)

A comprehensive report issued in 2018 began with the following statement: "Poor people in all parts of the world live and die with little or no palliative care or pain relief. Staring into this access abyss, one sees the depth of extreme suffering in the cruel face of poverty and inequity." (21) The report details the limitations of morphine availability throughout the world and goes on to state: "The fact that access to such an inexpensive, essential, and effective intervention is denied to most patients in low-income and middle-income countries...and in particular to poor people — including many poor or otherwise vulnerable people in high-income countries — is a medical, public health, and moral failing, and a travesty of justice." (21)

Five billion people are estimated to live in countries with little or no access to pain relief. Limited availability, cost, and over-regulation of opioids are significant factors in the widespread suffering from unrelieved pain in much of the world. (18-21) Global health programs focus on extending life and productivity, using statistics on death and disability, but there is little emphasis on pain relief. As pointed out by Dr. Richard Horton, editor-in-chief of the medical journal *Lancet,* little attention has been given to the major problem of unrelieved pain and that "[p]alliative care and pain relief are some of the most neglected dimensions of global health today." (22) The *Annals of the*

New York Academy of Sciences published a plea to clinicians that they must fully utilize medications, including opioids, to reduce pain and suffering, especially for cancer patients. (23)

CHRONIC PAIN

Some individuals have pain which persists for long periods of time. When pain lasts more than three months, i.e., beyond the time that one would expect normal healing from an injury, it is classified as chronic pain. (24) Although this type of pain may be less severe than the types of pain described above, the nearly constant pain takes its toll on the individual's quality of life.

Unrelieved chronic pain is a problem worldwide. Studies have found that in a given year over 1/3 of people living in developed countries and more than 40% of people living in less developed countries experience chronic pain. (25, 26)

Chronic pain is widespread in the US. A 2018 report by the Centers for Disease Control and Prevention (CDC) estimates that 20% of US adults live with chronic pain, ranging from patients with mild pain, who take daily over-the-counter pain medicines, to cancer patients who are dying with excruciating pain. (27) The CDC suggests that this percentage is likely an under-estimate, since their study did not include children or people living in nursing homes. (27) The percentage also varies widely in subgroups of the population, depending on income, age, and level of education. (27-28) Economic costs of pain are enormous. The total annual cost of pain in the US, including direct health care costs, loss of productivity and disability costs has been estimated between $560 and $635 billion. (27, 29)

The elderly in particular often suffer from chronic pain. Up to 50% of non-hospitalized adults over the age of 65 have some type of chronic pain. (30, 31) Moreover, the older the individual, the less likely he will receive appropriate pain medications. (30-32) Under-utilization of opioids is considered to be one cause of unrelieved chronic pain in the elderly, even for cancer patients. (32, 33)

Chronic pain is endemic among nursing home residents. (30, 34, 35) In one study, 66% of nursing home residents had chronic pain, but half the time the treating physicians did not detect the problem. (30, 34) A 2015 study of over 8,000 nursing home residents found that many cancer patients with nearly constant pain had not received any pain-relieving medications. (36) This report prompted an editorial entitled "Pain Management in American Nursing Homes – A Long Way to Go." (37) Clearly, some of the most vulnerable people in our society continue to suffer needlessly from pain!

Pain has enormous social impact. Chronic pain limits the ability to work and greatly diminishes quality of life. People in pain often decrease their physical activity, resulting in loss of muscle strength and further disability. Depressed mood is common among pain patients, leading to fewer social interactions and a lower level of engagement in activities which previously brought pleasure and happiness. Unrelieved chronic pain can lead to suicide. It has been estimated that between 5-14% of people with chronic pain actually attempt suicide. (38) A recent in-depth study of the medical records of more than 120,000 people who died by suicide found that 8.8% had chronic pain. (39) The authors suggest that these numbers likely represent an underestimation of the suicide rate by people with chronic pain, due to limitations on availability of data. More than half of the chronic pain patients who committed suicide died from gun-related injuries, whereas 16% died from an opioid overdose. (39)

Low Back Pain

Among the many types of chronic pain, low back pain is one of the most common and is a major cause of disability. (40-42) It has been estimated that 80% of adults in the US experience low back pain at some time in their lives. (42) Most patients with low back pain do recover within a relatively short time, since normal connective tissues usually heal within 6-12 weeks. However, in some patients the pain persists.

Chronic low back pain (cLBP) has a major socioeconomic impact. This single type of chronic pain has been reported to be the 3rd most expensive medical problem in the US (after cancer and cardiovascular disease), the 5th most common reason for hospitalization and the 3rd most frequent reason for a surgical procedure. (41, 42) cLBP is the most common cause of disability in the US for individuals younger than 45 years. Each year, 3-4% of the US population is disabled due to cLBP, with up to 1% of the working-age US population permanently disabled. (42)

It is often difficult to determine the cause of cLBP. In some cases, inflammation may play a role. Many structures in the spine could be involved. cLBP is sometimes considered to be a degenerative condition, but often there is little correlation between radiological signs of spinal degeneration and the painful symptoms. (43-46)

Osteoarthritis Pain

Osteoarthritis (OA) is another common type of chronic pain and a significant cause of disability. OA is typified by joint pain, often persistent knee pain. One study estimated that in a one-year period, ~25% of people over the age of 55 have an episode of persistent knee pain. (47) Other major sites are hands, spine, and hips. The prevalence of OA is expected to increase as the overall population ages.

There is no cure for OA, since the underlying joint damage can't be reversed. Treatment is directed at reducing pain and improving function of the affected joints. Mild OA pain can often be relieved through exercise, weight loss, and more appropriate shoes. Multiple types of the medications described in Chapter 6 are used to relieve OA pain. Replacement of a knee or hip joint is considered only when medications do not relieve debilitating pain or improve everyday functions, such as walking and sleeping. (48)

Fibromyalgia

Another major type of chronic pain is fibromyalgia (FM), which is characterized by persistent widespread musculoskeletal pain, along with fatigue, sleep disturbance, decreased ability to concentrate, impaired memory, and other symptoms. Individuals with FM feel intense pain in response to stimuli which most people would find either non-painful or only mildly painful. A diagnosis of FM is often given when there is no readily identifiable cause of the chronic musculoskeletal pain, along with the other symptoms. (49) Approximately 3% of females in the US have fibromyalgia; the prevalence is much lower in men (0.5%).

Historically, FM has been one of the most misunderstood painful conditions. The symptoms have been attributed to a variety of causes. In the late 19th century, this disorder was considered to be a psychiatric or psychosomatic disease because the patients did not have any obvious pathology in their muscles or other tissues. The term fibromyalgia was not widely used until the 1970s. (49) Even today, many patients with FM are misdiagnosed due to poor understanding of the pathology.

However, knowledge about FM has increased substantially in recent years. (49, 50) It is now considered to be a neurosensory disorder, meaning that a variety of abnormalities exist in the nervous system, including abnormalities in pain processing. In FM, the central nervous system (CNS), which includes the spinal cord and the brain, becomes "sensitized," so that the CNS amplifies the sensation of pain. (49, 50) FM is often characterized by abnormal levels of both excitatory and inhibitory neurotransmitters. (49, 50) (see Chapter 1, Table 3.) There appears to be a genetic component in FM, since first-degree relatives have an eightfold greater risk of developing FM than rheumatoid arthritis. (51) Psychological factors do play a role, but it is now widely accepted that FM is not a psychiatric disorder. In a recent review, Helen Cohen argues that a multidisciplinary approach is needed to treat FM, using non-pharmacologic therapies, patient education, and medications as needed to help control symptoms. (50)

Neuropathic Pain

Neuropathic pain is a type of chronic pain which is especially difficult to relieve. Neuropathic pain results from damage to nerves, which can occur after a traumatic injury or surgery. Certain diseases can also lead to neuropathic pain. The pain, which is often described as burning, electric, or shooting, can be quite severe and last for an extended period of time. In some cases, the pain eventually disappears, whereas in other cases the pain continues for a lifetime. The prevalence of neuropathic pain has been estimated between 1% and 7% of the general population. It is more common in women than men and in people over fifty years of age. (52, 53)

Post-herpetic neuralgia, which can develop in individuals who had chicken pox many years earlier, is one type of neuropathic pain. The virus which causes chicken pox can lie dormant in the individual's nerves for many years, but then become reactivated. The reactivated virus first produces a characteristic rash known as shingles or *herpes zoster*. The rash from the acute infection is often painful. But after the rash has healed, many patients develop neuropathic pain. Development of chronic neuropathic pain is more common with advancing age; 48% of patients ages 70-79 who had shingles experience pain lasting longer than a year. (54)

Many cancer patients develop a type of neuropathic pain following chemotherapy. Up to 1/3 of cancer patients who are considered cured or in remission have chronic pain resulting from the treatment they received. The pain often decreases with time, but many former cancer patients continue to suffer from neuropathic pain six months later. (55)

People with diabetes often develop neuropathic pain, which

is most pronounced in the legs. After many years of poor glucose control, up to half of people with diabetes have neuropathic pain. Patients with HIV/AIDS commonly have neuropathic pain. Spinal cord injury and other conditions which affect the nervous system can also lead to neuropathic pain. (54)

PAIN MANAGEMENT IN INFANTS AND CHILDREN

The turn of the 21st century did bring some improvements in pediatric pain management, especially for older children. The editors of a textbook entitled *Pain in Infants, Children and Adolescents* noted that substantial changes in pediatric pain management had occurred between publication of two editions of the book in 1993 and 2003. (56, 57) Over this period of ten years, new research had altered views about pain in infants and resulted in changes in clinical practice. Moreover, the public began to demand more aggressive and effective pain management for infants and children. The 2003 edition stated that, by this time, most children in the hospital were receiving adequate pain control after surgery, but that pain management was still a significant problem in infants and very young children with chronic diseases or following outpatient surgery. (57) The editors concluded that many infants and young children were still suffering needlessly from unrelieved pain. (57, 58) A clinical research study published in 2003 found that children under age two still received fewer pain-relieving medications than older children, in spite of having conditions which generated substantial pain. (59)

Neonates

The American Academy of Pediatrics (AAP) and the Canadian Paediatric Society published a joint policy statement in 2006, pointing out that both modern medicine and parents' expectations were now calling for better pain prevention and relief for neonates. (60)

Of course, it is difficult to determine whether a very young pre-ver-
bal child is in pain, but this 2006 policy statement concluded that
methods to reduce pain were still underutilized during the many
pain-inducing procedures that neonates typically undergo. (60-62)
Even a decade later in 2016, an updated AAP policy stated that
"proven and safe therapies are currently underused for routine minor, yet painful procedures" in neonates. (63)

The 2016 AAP policy statement discussed both medications and
non-medicinal methods to reduce pain in neonates. The non-medicinal methods included concurrent breastfeeding or administration of
a sweet oral solution during painful procedures. Evidence was presented that a sweet solution could be effective in reducing mild or
moderate procedural pain in infants. (63) A subsequent extensive
review of multiple studies also concluded that an oral sucrose solution can reduce pain in neonates. (64) I remind you, dear reader,
about the statement I mentioned in Chapter 3, which said that simply providing sugar water could adequately prevent pain in infants
undergoing surgery! (65) This statement was from a book published
in 1938. Of course, it would be unethical today to perform surgery on
infants without anesthesia, and no doubt your first reaction to the
1938 statement was that this was barbaric and certainly no longer
valid in the 21st century. Nevertheless, the 2016 and 2017 publications *do* support the use of sweet solutions, combined with other
methods, to help reduce infants' pain during *minorly* painful procedures, such as venipuncture, heel lance, and injections. As in many
areas of medicine, recent research has confirmed that some older
methods to reduce pain indeed do have some degree of validity.

Children in Emergency Departments

Many older children experience broken limbs resulting from
sports or rough play and typically go to an emergency department.
A 1995 study of emergency departments in Illinois hospitals found

that only 50% of children experiencing moderate to severe pain due to a broken bone were offered a pain-relieving medication. (66) Even in 2015, only 32% of children with documented pain received either a medicinal or non-medicinal treatment to relieve their pain in the emergency room of one suburban Chicago hospital. (67)

Inadequate pain relief for children in emergency departments is certainly not limited to the US. A 2016 study of an emergency department in Norway involved 243 children (ages 3-15) and multiple physicians. In this study, each child's pain was assessed not only by the physician, but also by the child himself. Based on the doctor's assessment of pain severity, pain medications were provided to only 42% of the children with severe pain. Unfortunately, pain relief was even worse based on the children's own reports of their pain; pain-relieving medications were provided to only 14% of the children who said themselves that they were in severe pain. As with many other studies described in this book, it appeared that the doctors had consistently and significantly underestimated the pain actually experienced by the children. (68)

Hospitalized Children

Although pain relief for pediatric inpatients has improved (57), some other studies report that pain relief for hospitalized children is still woefully inadequate. (69, 70) For example, one report from 2014 found that 86% of hospitalized children experienced pain, with 40% having moderate to severe pain. (70) Disturbingly, physicians often did not document the children's pain in the medical records. (69, 70)

RACIAL DISPARITIES IN PAIN MANAGEMENT IN THE UNITED STATES

More than 150 years after the Civil War, the United States is still highly segregated. Both overt and subtle racial discrimination exist in many spheres of modern society, including health care.

Multiple studies have shown striking differences in prescribing patterns of pain medications to black *vs* white patients. The National Hospital Ambulatory Medical Care Survey, which included more than 65,000 patients, found that white patients with migraines or low back pain were much more likely to receive an analgesic in emergency departments than black patients. (71) Moreover, among the patients with back pain who did receive an analgesic, twice as many whites as blacks were given an opioid medication. When physicians had to rely only upon the patient's own report of his migraine or back pain, significant racial bias occurred. In contrast, such racial disparities did not exist when the patients had broken bones. Physicians then prescribed analgesics similarly for these white and black patients who had an obvious cause of pain. (71)

Another study, which evaluated patterns of opioid prescribing from 1993 to 2005, found even greater racial bias. In this study, fewer black patients received opioids than white patients in emergency departments, even when there was an obvious cause of pain such as a broken bone. This disparity between white and black patients also existed between white and Hispanic or Asian patients. The racial disparities in opioid prescribing did not diminish over this twelve year time period. (72) A later study published in 2012 found similar disparity in opioid-prescribing patterns for black vs white pain patients (73), in spite of overall increased emphasis on pain relief at this time. Examination of health records between 2011 and 2014 for over 8000 patients from multiple Community Health Centers in Connecticut also revealed racial disparity in treating both severe acute and chronic pain, even though these health centers had specific mandates to reduce such disparities. White patients received approximately twice as many opioid prescriptions as Hispanic patients and approximately 50% more than black patients. (74)

Pharmacies also may exhibit racial bias. For example, pharmacies in areas with primarily minority populations were much less likely to have sufficient opioid analgesics in stock than pharmacies in predominantly white areas. (75, 76) Black patients who received opioids for pain relief at a US Veteran's Administration Healthcare pharmacy were subjected to more monitoring with urine tests than white patients, were less likely to be referred to a pain specialist and were more likely to be assessed for possible substance abuse. (77)

Attitudes among recent medical students and medical residents suggest that racial bias is not going to disappear with younger doctors. A substantial number of white medical students and residents wrongly believe that black and white patients have biological differences in pain perception and that blacks experience less pain than whites. (78) Certainly, such misconceptions can contribute to racial bias and the widespread under treatment of pain in black people.

DIMINISHED EMPHASIS ON PAIN RELIEF IN THE 21ST CENTURY

As described in the first part of this chapter, unrelieved pain continues to be a major medical problem for people in multiple settings and the result of many conditions. The rest of this chapter discusses some of the reasons for the continuing problem of pain in the 21st century.

The importance of pain relief gained greater recognition in the latter part of the 20th century (see Chapter 3). At that time, health care providers were more likely to take a patient's self-reported pain seriously and prescribe pain-relieving medications, including the strong opioids. But there was an unexpected consequence. As prescriptions for strong opioids increased substantially, the abuse of opioids reached crisis proportion, especially in the US. As a result, health care providers in the 21st century have become reluctant to prescribe opioids for pain relief (see Chapter 7). I argue that the opioid crisis has led to an overall devaluing of effective pain relief.

For example, delegates at the 2016 Congress of the American Academy of Family Physicians (AAFP) voted to remove pain as the 5th vital sign when assessing a patient's health status. (79) A later survey found that nearly half of physicians and nurses strongly agreed with the AAFP recommendation that pain should no longer be considered the 5th vital sign. (80) The House of Delegates of the American Medical Association (AMA) also voted to eliminate pain as a vital sign. (79)

Agencies and commissions in the US Federal Government also appear to be devaluing pain relief. The President's Commission on Combating Drug Addiction and the Opioid Crisis issued a report in late 2017, calling for removal of pain as a vital sign in new federal policies. (81)

Another example comes from the Centers for Medicare and Medicaid Services (CMS) which asks patients to complete a survey when they leave the hospital. In the past, the overall score of this survey has been used by the CMS as one of the criteria to determine the how much the hospitals are reimbursed for patient care. (82) Three of the questions on the survey ask the patients how well their pain was controlled while in the hospital. However, these questions about pain control have become controversial. Some people believe that the questions pressure physicians to prescribe more opioids in order to improve scores on the surveys, and therefore increase hospital revenue.

In April 2016, a letter signed by 58 distinguished physicians who specialize in pain management or addiction treatment was sent to the CMS. The letter asked that the pain-related questions be removed from the survey. The American Pain Society and some other societies countered by stating that the CMS should retain these questions; their position was that removing the questions would be a step back to an earlier time when pain control was not considered to be very important. As a compromise, the CMS decided to retain the questions in modified forms, but to eliminate them from the calculation of reimbursement to hospitals. (82) Although certainly less than if the questions about pain control had been completely removed, the compromise did diminish emphasis on pain relief.

PAIN CANNOT BE MEASURED OBJECTIVELY

A major reason that pain is not adequately treated today and even undervalued by some health care providers is that there is no objective way to measure pain. This is in contrast with many other medical conditions. For example, high blood pressure (hypertension) is readily diagnosed since it can be easily measured through routine use of blood pressure cuffs in physicians' offices and pharmacies. Similarly, diabetes can be diagnosed through measurement of glucose and another molecule known as HbA1C in blood. But currently there is no objective method for health care providers to accurately determine how much pain a patient is actually experiencing.

Today, a health care provider may ask the patient directly about his pain, including its severity. Several pain scales have been developed that rely on the patient's self-report of pain. The most commonly used is the Visual Analog Scale (VAS), which has several forms. One form uses a scale in which the patient is asked to describe his pain with a number ranging from 0 (no pain) to 10 (the most severe pain imaginable). Another form has a series of faces which range from a happy face, depicting no pain, to faces which are frowning, crying, etc. to express varying pain levels. This scale is particularly useful for small children or patients with limited cognitive abilities. Another scale is the McGill Pain Scale which asks patients to describe their pain, using words such as "throbbing," "stabbing," "dull," and "shooting." Although some clinicians have found these descriptors helpful in diagnosis, the McGill Pain Scale is not widely utilized today.

All pain scales rely on the patient's own description of his pain. But often the health care provider questions whether the pain level is truly what the patient says is it is. The lack of an objective measure of pain can cause a discrepancy between the severity of pain reported by the patient and that assessed by the clinician. There can be distrust and misunderstanding between patients and their families or physicians regarding the severity or even the existence of the pain.

A review of eighty studies conducted between 1991 and 2016 found that the estimation of a patient's pain by health care professionals was consistently lower than the patient's own reported pain. (83) Underestimation occurred in 78% of these studies, which included hospital settings, primary care, nursing homes, and out-patients. Disturbingly, the underestimation was greatest with the most severe pain. Unfortunately, there was no indication that the situation was improving over this twenty-five-year time period. (83)

In an interesting study, health care providers were asked to rate the severity of pain in patients based on videos of the patients, along with any existing medical evidence to support a pain diagnosis. Overall, in spite of the patients' self-reported pain, the health care providers rated the pain severity lower when medical evidence was not present. In addition, these patients received less sympathy and help. Moreover, when psychosocial situations were present, patients were less likely to have their self-reported pain taken seriously by a medical professional. (84)

A review of multiple published studies evaluated whether cancer patients received adequate pain-relieving medications. (85) This review compared the patient's own reported level of pain with the type and strength of pain-relieving medications provided to the patient. Results from this analysis demonstrated a low level of congruence between the pain severity and the type of medication prescribed; 43% of the cancer patients had not received medications which would have provided adequate pain relief. (85) It is likely that underestimation of the patients' pain by the health care providers played a major role in the undertreatment.

In addition to the discrepancy between the *level* of pain reported by the patient and that assessed by the health care provider, sometimes the health care providers even doubt the *existence* of the reported pain. This is especially the case when a physical examination does not provide a medical explanation for the reported pain. A patient may be viewed as imagining the pain or even falsely claiming to be in pain.

When a patient reports having severe pain, but the physician does not find any serious issues in a routine physical exam or follow-up imaging, the physician faces a dilemma. Does the physician accept the patient's self-reported pain and prescribe pain-relieving medications, or instead conclude that the patient is not truly in pain and rather is "drug-seeking"? A recent study interviewed a varied group of physicians about this issue. (86) The following are excerpts from the publication, including direct quotes from some of the physicians who were interviewed. "[P]hysicians reported skepticism about the value of patient self-reported pain....Physicians expressed concern about the inconsistency of self-reported pain, observed behaviors, and exam findings. For example: Somebody will say 'Oh, I have a ten out of [ten] pain,' but they're sitting there, comfortably. They're walking around, totally fine, and you're like, 'This is not what I would consider ten out of ten pain'....Similarly another physician expressed frustration about the legitimacy of pain presentations that are inconsistent with physical exam: 'A lot of people come in with this chronic back pain that – it should present one way but they're in pain all over the place. Their pain is just completely ridiculous, out of proportion to exam. You just barely touch them....Jumping off the table – you know it like, all right, it's probably not real'." (86) The authors of another study found that clinicians tended to "assign greater weight to non-verbal expressions [of pain] than to patients' self-report." The authors concluded that there are "markers of deception" which physicians can utilize to determine when people are lying about their pain. (87)

Nearly one-third of claims about chronic pain in lawsuits involving personal injury or disability were judged to be "probable malingering." (88) Of course, it is likely that some of these claims were dishonest. Nevertheless, since it is not currently possible to objectively determine the validity and severity of many claims regarding chronic pain, distrust can exacerbate the problem of unrelieved pain.

One publication concludes that "some primary care physicians actively avoid caring for chronic non-cancer pain. Given the enormous prevalence of chronic pain....this finding raises serious concerns about patients' access to effective chronic non-cancer pain care." (86) Clearly, new methods are needed to objectively determine pain severity so that people truly in pain can receive needed relief. This is discussed further in Chapter 10.

RELUCTANCE OF PATIENTS TO USE PAIN-RELIEVING MEDICATIONS

There are many reasons why people are often reluctant to use modern pain-relieving medications. Some people prefer to first try herbal products, other types of traditional medicine, or some of the alternative methods described in Chapter 9. Sometimes people in the hospital, who want to be viewed as "good patients" and not a "bother" to nursing staff or other caregivers, do not admit the severity of their pain or request pain relief. Other patients fear that if they get pain relief now, the medications will no longer be effective if the pain becomes worse later.

Cancer patients with moderate to severe pain who did not want to use the prescribed analgesics were asked why they were reluctant to use the pain medications. Some patients said they felt that all medications should be avoided because they are "toxins." Other patients replied that clinicians or family members had previously stigmatized them for their use of analgesics, especially opioids. (89)

Much of the general populace today is afraid to use opioids prescribed by their physicians for relief of severe pain. They have been told by well-meaning people that they should not use the prescribed opioids due to fear of addiction. However, when the medications are appropriately taken under a doctor's supervision for pain relief, the chances of addiction are less than commonly thought, as discussed in Chapter 7. Physicians, pharmacists, or other health care professionals may also unwittingly give the impression that it is wrong to take opioids to relieve pain.

I remember visiting a dear family member in the hospital. He was over ninety years old and had just had his leg amputated due to severe circulation problems. As I talked with him, he stated in a very hushed tone that his IV drip contained morphine. He clearly was concerned about receiving opioids to relieve his pain. I reassured him that it was okay to take morphine to relieve his pain. All people need to be reminded that being in pain does not make them better persons, but rather that relief of pain is good for them.

Another close member of my family was recently prescribed hydrocodone to relieve her severe pain. Although the woman is over ninety years old and her mental faculties are fully intact, one of her sons feared that she would become addicted. As a result, he indicated that he was going to hide the medication so she would not use it!

PAIN EDUCATION HAS BEEN LIMITED

Patients themselves often do not have adequate information about pain. Among Americans who rated their pain as severe or unbearable, 18% had not visited a health care professional, because they did not think that anything could be done to relieve their suffering. (90, 91)

Although nurses are the front-line caregivers for patients in pain, education of nurses about pain and pain management was very limited in the past. A chapter entitled "Principles of Medical Nursing" in a 1932 textbook for nursing students contained only three pages about pain. The pain-relieving methods described were limiting movement of the patient and use of cold or hot applications. The only mention of medications to relieve pain was a single sentence in the introduction to the book. (92)

Somewhat later, a 1960 nursing textbook on care of surgical patients emphasized preventing complications through proper positioning of the patient and the importance of coughing to relieve lung congestion. (93) There were only a couple sentences about relief of post-surgical pain. These sentences stated that opioids could be used cautiously, but their real purpose was to enable the patients to cough and breathe more deeply when they were in less pain. (93) Pain relief itself was given little consideration. The index to this textbook contained only a single reference to morphine, which stated that it can be used to quiet the patient in preparation for surgery. (93)

Even by 2000, a review of fifty major nursing textbooks reported that only 0.5% of the books' content discussed pain. (94) None of these textbooks provided guidance on titration of opioids, although nurses frequently make titration decisions. Instead of emphasizing how to use opioids safely, the textbooks focused on opioid side effects. (94) Non-pharmacological approaches to relieve pain received approximately twice the coverage of analgesic medications. Overall, the language in the textbooks implied that use of medications should be avoided or at least minimized. One conclusion from the review of these textbooks was that the ongoing problem of inadequate pain relief is "related to failure to use analgesics." (94)

Most doctors also have inadequate knowledge about pain and pain relief. In spite of the prevalence of pain and the resulting suffering and disability, medical schools have provided only limited education about pain. Analysis of two major pediatric medical textbooks found that pain was only mentioned in a few places and then only in the context of its role in diagnosis of a particular disease. (95-97) A 2011 evaluation of pain education in 117 medical schools in US and Canada concluded that "pain education for North American medical students is limited, variable, and often fragmentary." (98)

The Johns Hopkins University School of Medicine has developed a new course on Pain Care Medicine that is now required for their first-year medical students. (99) Their website states that when this course was developed in 2010, only ~10% of US medical schools included pain management education. However, it is likely that most other medical schools have followed suit, by also adding courses about pain and pain relief to the curriculum.

In 2013 the influential American Medical Association (AMA) developed a new continuing medication education program, specifically on pain management, for physicians. A past president of the AMA stated in an interview that "Revisions to this education program will help physicians maintain an understanding of appropriate pain management and ensure legitimate patients get the treatment they need while helping to prevent prescription drug abuse and diversion." (100)

CONCLUSION

Although there have been major advancements in many other areas of medicine, unrelieved pain continues to be a significant problem. Most types of chronic pain, and even acute pain, are often not adequately relieved.

Several factors contribute to widespread unrelieved pain. These include lack of an objective way for physicians to assess pain, as well as inadequate education about pain. Moreover, the current opioid abuse crisis is now reducing an emphasis on the importance of pain relief. In addition to the factors discussed in this chapter, understanding of the science and medicine of pain lags behind that of many other medical conditions. In particular, none of the current methods adequately relieve many types of pain. The next chapters discuss the uses, the limitations, and the science of both current medications and alternative methods to relieve pain.

CHAPTER 6

HOW GOOD ARE
CURRENT MEDICATIONS
IN RELIEVING PAIN?

As described in Chapter 1, there are several types of pain. However, to discuss pain medications, it is useful to classify most types of pain into two broad categories: *neuropathic and non-neuropathic*. In general, different medications are used to relieve these two types of pain. Medications discussed in this chapter can relieve pain to varying degrees, but none is risk-free. Although the risks of opioids are well-known, commonly used over-the-counter medications to relieve pain also have risks.

MEDICATIONS FOR NON-NEUROPATHIC PAIN

Most current medications to relieve non-neuropathic pain fall into two distinct groups. One group consists of non-opioid medications, such as the non-steroidal anti-inflammatory drugs (NSAIDs) and acetaminophen. NSAIDs include aspirin, ibuprofen, celecoxib, and naproxen, which all have a similar biochemical mechanism of action. The second group consists of the opioids, including tramadol, morphine, fentanyl, oxycodone, and hydrocodone. Both groups of medications originated with plant extracts that had been used for centuries or even millennia for pain relief.

The World Health Organization (WHO) has established a guideline, known as the three-step "analgesic ladder," for management of non-neuropathic pain (Table 1). (1) In this guideline, originally developed to manage pain in cancer patients, pain is differentiated according to its severity. Recommended medications are given for each level of pain. For mild pain, medications such as aspirin, ibuprofen, or acetaminophen are recommended. For more intense pain, a weak opioid such as codeine or tramadol may be needed, often in combination with a Step 1 medication. For severe pain, strong opioids such as morphine are required. Other medications, which are not specifically pain drugs but rather are known as adjuvant drugs, can be added to help reduce pain at all levels of severity. (1)

Table 1. WHO Pain Relief Ladder

Step 1. Mild pain	
Non-Opioid Analgesics	Non-steroidal anti-inflammatory drugs (NSAIDS) Aspirin Ibuprofen Acetaminophen
Step 2. Moderate pain	
Weak Opioids	Codeine, Tramadol
Step 3. Severe pain	
Strong Opioids	Morphine, Oxycodone, Hydromorphone, Fentanyl

Adapted from the WHO 3-Step Analgesic Ladder (1)

Non-Steroidal Anti-Inflammatory Drugs (NSAIDs)

The most widely known member of the NSAID class is aspirin, which has a long and interesting history. Over 2000 years ago, extracts prepared from the bark of willow trees were used to treat pain and inflammation. These extracts were the forerunner of modern-day aspirin. Hippocrates (440-377 BCE), Dioscorides, Pliny the Elder and Galen (1st and 2nd centuries CE) described the therapeutic properties of the bark and leaves of willow trees. (2) Indeed, many cultures over the last two millennia utilized the pain-relieving effects of willow bark extracts. (2)

Plant extracts have been used since antiquity for the treatment of a variety of human ailments, not only pain. Natural product extracts are available today in over-the-counter products in drug stores and health food stores. Such extracts usually consist of multiple compounds, which vary depending on how the extract has been prepared. In contrast, prescription drugs and most over-the-counter drugs consist of well-defined pure compounds. In order to have consistency in effectiveness and safety, it is necessary to know both the specific ingredients and their amounts in a medication.

In 1763 Edward Stone at the University of Oxford identified the main pain-relieving ingredient in willow bark extracts. (3) Dr. Stone called this compound salicylic acid, based on the Latin word *salix* for the willow tree. More than 100 years later, the chemists Felix Hoffmann and Arthur Eichengrün, who were working in the pharmaceutical laboratory of the German company Friedrich Bayer & Co, modified the compound to yield acetylsalicylic acid, which is the modern medication known as aspirin. (4, 5) Subsequently, the Bayer Company demonstrated the clinical utility of acetylsalicylic acid for treating pain and inflammation and began marketing their branded Bayer's Aspirin™ in 1899. (4,5) Today, Bayer continues to market it under the brand name

Genuine Bayer® Aspirin. Aspirin is also available as a generic drug, manufactured and marketed by multiple companies.

Aspirin is a widely used medication today, and it is likely that most people have taken aspirin to relieve minor pain. Ibuprofen is another member of the NSAID class commonly used to treat pain and inflammation. Ibuprofen is sold as a generic drug but is also the main ingredient in brands such as *Motrin®* and *Advil®*. Both aspirin and ibuprofen are widely available without a prescription but the drugs are not risk-free. Long-term use of high doses or even relatively modest doses of either drug can have a significant side effect, specifically bleeding in the gastrointestinal (GI) tract. This bleeding in the stomach and intestines can be quite severe and even fatal. The American College of Gastroenterology has highlighted the GI risks of NSAIDs and published guidelines for their use. (6) These guidelines point out that GI bleeding from long term use of NSAIDs leads to the hospitalization of 100,000 patients per year in the US, with up to 10,000 deaths. (6)

How Do NSAIDs Relieve Pain but Also Cause Side Effects?

It has been known since the early 1970s that NSAIDs inhibit the body's formation of molecules known as prostaglandins, which play an important role in pain and inflammation. When NSAIDs decrease the level of prostaglandins, pain and inflammation are reduced. However, prostaglandins also play an important role in maintaining a protective barrier in several internal organs, including the stomach and kidneys. By decreasing the level of prostaglandins, aspirin and ibuprofen threaten this protective barrier and, in particular, increase the risk of GI bleeding.

NSAIDs decrease prostaglandin formation by inhibiting an enzyme known as cyclooxygenase (COX). In the 1990's, scientists discovered that the COX enzyme exists in at least two forms, known as COX-1 and COX-2. Moreover, the two forms of the COX enzyme were found to be active under different conditions and distributed differently in various organs in the body. COX-2 was reported to be active primarily during an inflammatory response, whereas COX-1 was continuously active, especially in the GI tract. These discoveries caused considerable excitement in the scientific community since they were thought to provide opportunities to develop a safer NSAID. The hypothesis was that a *selective* drug, which preferentially blocked the activity of COX-2 but maintained COX-1 activity, would continue to have the pain-relieving effects of aspirin and ibuprofen, but would preserve the protective barrier in internal organs and reduce GI side effects. (7)

Indeed, as a result of these scientific discoveries, new drugs were developed which did preferentially inhibit COX-2 over COX-1. These new COX-2 inhibitors became known as rofecoxib (*Vioxx*™) and celecoxib (*Celebrex*™). Both were immediately hailed as important new ways to treat minor pains and inflammation without the GI safety concerns associated with aspirin and ibuprofen. As predicted, the new COX-2 inhibitors did retain the pain-relieving activities of aspirin and ibuprofen, and also reduced the risk of GI bleeding. (7)

However, the story turned out to be more complicated, since the COX-2 selective drugs did not have clearly superior safety profiles. (8) Troubling information began to emerge as more people began to use these new medications to relieve pain. Unfortunately, the selective COX-2 inhibitors appeared to be associated with serious cardiovascular (CV) side effects, including heart attacks and strokes. (8-10) Just as COX-1 plays a protective role in the GI tract, COX-2 was found to play a protective role in the heart. As a result, selectively inhibiting COX-2 could have detrimental CV side effects.

One of these new COX-2 selective drugs (*Vioxx*™) was voluntarily removed from the marketplace in 2004 due to the potential risk of heart attacks and strokes. The other COX-2 selective drug, known as celecoxib or *Celebrex*™, is still available and widely used, although the FDA requires a warning label about possible CV side effects.

However, we now know that the potential CV side effects are not limited to COX-2-selective medicines, but are also concerns with the non-selective NSAIDs. (10-13) In 2015 the FDA mandated that labels on all NSAIDs (except aspirin) must contain stronger warnings about CV risks. (12) The increased risk of heart attacks and strokes has been estimated to be between 10% and >50%, depending on the specific NSAID and the dose. (11) Unfortunately, scientists have not yet found a clear relationship between COX-2 selectivity and CV side effects. Two FDA advisory panels in 2018 have concluded that the CV safety of the COX-2 selective *Celebrex*™ is similar to that of non-selective NSAIDs such as ibuprofen. (14) In addition to concerns about possible CV side effects, prolonged use of NSAIDs may result in chronic kidney disease, consistent with the protective role of prostaglandins in many internal organs. (11)

Because most NSAIDs are available over the counter without a prescription, people often conclude that these medications are risk-free. As a result, people may not heed the warnings on the labels and take amounts of NSAIDs above the daily dosing limit. (15, 16) Due to the risks, some physicians have suggested that all NSAIDs should be available only by prescription. (16)

So, as with all medications, the pain-relieving benefits of NSAIDs must be weighed versus their risks. Most people who use NSAIDs to relieve mild pain do not experience serious side effects. Nevertheless, it must be remembered that NSAIDs are not risk-free, especially with long-term use.

Acetaminophen

Acetaminophen is another medication commonly used to treat minor pain. It is sold as a generic drug and also under the brand name *Tylenol*™. Outside the US, the generic name of this drug is paracetamol. Although acetaminophen is often used interchangeably with ibuprofen or other NSAIDs for pain relief, it does not have anti-inflammatory activity and therefore is not an NSAID. The biochemical mechanism by which acetaminophen relieves pain is not well understood. (17)

Acetaminophen does not appear to have the potential CV, GI, and kidney side effects associated with NSAIDs. However, acetaminophen is also not risk-free. High doses carry the risk of acute liver failure. As a result, the FDA has issued guidelines restricting the daily dose of acetaminophen. (18) Of particular concern is the presence of acetaminophen in many cold medications. Dangerous levels of acetaminophen can easily be reached by taking acetaminophen itself to relieve pain, along with other medications containing acetaminophen to treat symptoms of a cold. Labels of over-the-counter medications should be carefully scrutinized prior to taking both acetaminophen and cold medications.

Opioids

Opioids constitute the second major class of medications to relieve non-neuropathic pain. The use of opioids to relieve pain has a long history. Similar to aspirin, the history of opioids originates with extracts of a plant, in this case the poppy. Extracts from poppies, known as opium, were used to relieve pain in the ancient world. Centuries later, Arabic traders introduced opium to physicians in Europe. But by the 14th century, use of opium essentially disappeared in Europe when the bubonic plague was raging. Since the plague was considered to have originated in the East, perhaps

Europeans at this time feared anything associated with Eastern medicine. (19)

Opium was reintroduced to Europe in the 16th century by the Swiss-German physician Paracelsus. (19) Somewhat later, the English physician Thomas Sydenham developed a medication known as laudanum, which contained opium, sherry, and several spices. Laudanum became widely used in the 17th century, especially in England, to relieve pain as discussed in Chapter 2. Sydenham praised the use of laudanum and in particular, spoke of the value of opium in treating a variety of ailments. (20, 21)

Prior to the 19th century, opium was extracted from poppies by a variety of techniques, yielding potions of varying effectiveness. But early in the 19th century, the German pharmacist Friedrich Wilhelm Serturner isolated a pure crystalline substance from the opium extracts. He called this substance *morphium*, based on the Latin name Morpheus given by Ovid to the god of dreams. (22, 23) Serturner led experiments in both animals and humans which demonstrated that this single substance could relieve pain as effectively as the crude opium extracts. (22) The isolation of pure *morphium* (morphine) meant that it was now possible to standardize both the purity and strength of this powerful drug. Subsequently, a variety of medicines containing morphine were produced by pharmacists and widely provided to patients.

However, as morphine became widely available in the 19th and 20th centuries and used by large numbers of people to relieve pain and treat other ailments, abuse of this potent drug became more common. It was not until 1970 that the US adopted the Controlled Substances Act to reduce illicit trafficking of opioids and other drugs that had abuse potential. This act specified five categories (schedules) of drugs, based on their abuse/addiction potential (Table 2).

Table 2. Classification of Controlled Substances (Adapted from ref 24)

Classification	Definition	Examples
Schedule I	Drugs with no currently accepted medical use and high potential for abuse	Heroin, Marijuana (Cannabis), LSD
Schedule II	Drugs with high potential for abuse, with use potentially leading to severe psychological or physical dependence	Morphine, Oxycodone, Hydrocodone, Hydromorphone, *Nucynta*™ (Tapentadol)
Schedule III	Drugs with moderate to low potential for physical or psychological dependence	*Tylenol*™ with codeine (Acetaminophen with codeine)
Schedule IV	Drugs with low potential for abuse and low risk of dependence	*Ultram*™ (Tramadol), *Valium*™ (Diazepam), *Ativan*™ (Lorazepam)
Schedule V	Drugs with lower potential for abuse than Schedule IV, including preparations containing limited quantities of some narcotics	*Robitussin AC*™ (contains codeine), *Lyrica*™ (Pregabalin)

Drugs in Schedules I-IV are known as controlled substances. Schedule I consists of drugs with the highest abuse potential and no known medicinal purpose, such as heroin. Currently, marijuana is also in Schedule I, although recent legalization of medical marijuana in some states suggests that it may need to be reclassified. The strong prescription opioids, such as morphine and oxycodone, are in Schedule II. Weaker opioids such as tramadol are in Schedule IV. There are specific regulations for manufacturing, distributing, and prescribing the drugs in each of these categories.

Although they can certainly be abused, the opioids in Schedule

II are very effective in relieving many types of pain. Currently, there are no other medications which are as effective as the strong opioids in relieving severe pain. The World Health Organization (WHO) said that opioids are "absolutely necessary" when pain is moderate to severe. (25) The United Nations Office on Drugs and Crime stated: "Opioid analgesics are essential for sufficient pain management." and that "the medical use of narcotic drugs continued to be indispensable for the relief of pain and suffering and that adequate provision must be made to ensure their availability for such purposes." (26)

How Do Opioids Relieve Pain?

All drugs exert their effects by interacting with specific molecules present in various parts of the body. These molecules are classified as receptors, enzymes, or ion channels. Opioids bind to specific receptors on the surface of nerve cells (neurons). In the spinal cord, opioid-receptor interactions inhibit the release of molecules known as neurotransmitters, which decrease excitability of other neurons and therefore decrease pain. Opioids also bind to receptors in several parts of the brain. A major site of action of opioids in the brain is a region called the periaqueductal grey (PAG). Binding of opioids to their receptors on cells in the PAG sends a signal from the brain back down to the spinal cord, further releasing other types of neurotransmitters which decrease pain sensation. (see Chapter 1)

MEDICATIONS FOR NEUROPATHIC PAIN

Neuropathic pain is pain that develops as a result of injury to nerves. Various diseases, surgical procedures, or other types of injuries can cause nerve damage and lead to chronic neuropathic pain.

The medications most commonly used to relieve neuropathic pain are different from those used for other types of pain. These include pills to be taken orally, patches to be applied to the painful area, and drugs which must be injected (Table 3).

Table 3. Medications Commonly Used to Relieve Neuropathic Pain.

Pills
Neurontin™ (Gabapentin)
Lyrica™ (Pregabalin)
Tricyclic Antidepressants
Amitriptyline
Desipramine
Nortriptyline
SNRIs
Duloxetine
Venlafaxine
Patches
Lidocaine patch
Qutenza™ (Capsaicin patch)
Butrans™ (Buprenorphine patch)
Injectables
Prialt™ (Ziconotide)
Botox™ (Botulinum toxin)

Oral Medications

The most widely prescribed medications currently used to alleviate neuropathic pain are oral medications that were first developed either to block the seizures associated with epilepsy or to alleviate depression. (27, 28)

Carbamazepine was the first anti-epileptic drug used to treat neuropathic pain. However, side effects and drug-drug interactions limited its use for pain relief. Today, two other drugs, which were also originally developed to block epileptic seizures, are routinely prescribed to relieve neuropathic pain. The first of these is gabapentin, which is sold under the brand name *Neurontin*™. A closely related newer compound is pregabalin (sold under the brand name *Lyrica*™). Both are used to relieve neuropathic pain, especially pain resulting from shingles or uncontrolled diabetes. These medications exert their effects by blocking a specific type of calcium ion channel found on neurons, thereby decreasing neuronal excitation. (29)

Several oral medications originally developed to treat clinical depression are also commonly prescribed for neuropathic pain. One class of these drugs developed in the 1960s consists of the tricyclic antidepressants. This group of drugs, which includes amitriptyline, desipramine, and nortriptyline, alter chemical signaling between brain cells by a variety of mechanisms. Although they can alleviate depression and neuropathic pain in some patients, they do have many side effects. (29)

Today, members of a newer class of antidepressants are often prescribed to alleviate neuropathic pain. Drugs in this class are known as serotonin norepinephrine reuptake inhibitors (SNRIs). As the name indicates, these drugs, which include duloxetine and venlafaxine, specifically block the reuptake of the neurotransmitters serotonin and norepinephrine back into neurons, thereby increasing their concentrations in the regions between neurons. The increased concentrations lead to more interactions with specific neuronal receptors, resulting in a series of events which may alleviate both depression and neuropathic pain. The older tricyclic antidepressants also increase the concentrations of serotonin and norepinephrine, but they have additional activities. The newer SNRIs are more specific and have fewer side effects than the older drugs, but they may also be less effective. (29)

Unfortunately, none of the oral medications in Table 3 provide much relief of neuropathic pain. A comprehensive review found that these medications had only modest effects at best. (30)

Nevertheless, this review concluded that one of these oral medications should be tried first for relief of neuropathic pain. (30)

Other medications are now being evaluated for neuropathic pain relief. One of these is ketamine, which is commonly used as an intravenous anesthetic. Lower doses are beginning to be used to relieve acute post-operative pain. (31) An oral formulation of ketamine is being used for treatment-resistant severe depression and is also undergoing studies for relief of neuropathic pain. (32) However, it should be noted that ketamine is potentially addictive and can be abused.

Patches

Patches applied externally to painful areas are sometimes used to relieve neuropathic pain. The most common patch contains lidocaine, which is an anesthetic that reduces the excitability of neurons. Lidocaine is the same drug injected locally by dentists to reduce pain during dental procedures.

Another type of patch to relieve neuropathic pain contains the compound capsaicin. It is capsaicin which generates the hot burning sensation that occurs when eating food containing chili peppers. Capsaicin also causes a burning sensation when it comes in contact with skin, eyes or other membranes. So you may ask, why in the world would one apply an agent that causes a burning sensation to skin that is already painful? The answer lies in the way that capsaicin works. After the initial burning sensation, capsaicin causes peripheral nerves to become desensitized, which means they no longer transmit a pain signal, thereby alleviating neuropathic pain.

Qutenza™ is a patch which contains 8% capsaicin. Qutenza™ has been shown to reduce neuropathic pain in diabetic patients, HIV patients, and patients who previously had shingles. A single 30-minute treatment with the patch provides ~30% pain relief, which lasts for several weeks. (33, 34) But not all patients like to use these patches since the capsaicin causes an initial burning sensation, although this can be reduced by prior application of a local anesthetic cream. However, the *Qutenza*™ patch is expensive; a single patch is currently selling for more than $800. Capsaicin is also available as a cream without a prescription. These creams, containing much lower amounts of capsaicin, cause little or no burning sensation but also do not provide much pain relief.

Another type of patch called *Butrans*™ contains the opioid buprenorphine. This patch has been approved by the FDA to relieve moderate to severe chronic pain. Buprenorphine is the same drug described in Chapter 7 to treat opioid addiction. In one study, buprenorphine patches reduced pain by a least 30% in most patients with painful diabetic neuropathy, although the side effects of nausea, vomiting, and constipation associated with opioids were common. (35) Generic forms of the buprenorphine patch are now available and are not overly expensive.

Injected Medications

Prialt™ is a relatively new drug to relieve severe chronic pain, especially neuropathic pain. This drug, also known as ziconotide, is a small peptide originally identified in the venom from a cone snail. It relieves pain by blocking nerves in the spinal cord that transfer the pain signal to the brain. However, it must be injected directly into the space around the spinal cord via an infusion pump. Due to this route of administration, *Prialt*™ is used only for people who have not received adequate pain relief from other medications. (36)

Botulinum neurotoxins block neuronal signaling through a variety of mechanisms, including inhibiting the release of neurotransmitters and inflammatory mediators from neurons. Botulinum toxin type A, which is marketed by Allergan as *Botox*™, is approved by the FDA for treating chronic migraine, in addition to its well-known cosmetic effects. Recent studies have found that *Botox* ™ (or other subtypes of botulinum toxin) can also alleviate neuropathic pain. One study has demonstrated that two series of botulinum toxin A injections at twelve-week intervals are safe and effective in reducing neuropathic pain, especially pain resulting from trauma or surgery. Botulinum injections are most effective in relieving pain that is localized to a specific highly sensitive area. Injections of botulinum toxins can also decrease pain in other types of neuropathic pain such as post-herpetic neuralgia, which can occur after an episode of shingles. (37)

MEDICATIONS FOR MIGRAINE

Migraine is a distinct neurological disorder. (38) Migraine headaches are generally believed to be caused by a combination of neuronal and vascular activities, causing dilation of blood vessels in the brain. But the relative importance of the nervous and vascular systems in the pathophysiology of migraine continues to be controversial. (39)

The triptans are the most common medications currently used to relieve migraine pain. They not only relieve pain but also help relieve other migraine symptoms such as nausea, vomiting, and extreme sensitivity to light or sound. Triptans selectively stimulate serotonin receptors on neurons in the brain and perhaps at other sites in the body. (40) It is generally believed that triptans cause contraction of muscles surrounding the blood vessels in the brain, thereby narrowing the blood vessels and relieving the symptoms of migraine. Sumatriptan (brand name *Imitrex*™) is the most well-known of the triptans.

Although the triptans are effective in relieving ongoing migraine headaches, they do not prevent headaches or reduce their number. Importantly, in 2018 the FDA approved a new drug which does effectively reduce the frequency of migraine attacks. (41) This medication is called *Aimovig*™ and is administered once a month by self-injection. (42) *Aimovig*™ acts in a different way from the triptans since it blocks the receptor for a peptide known as the calcitonin gene-related peptide (CGRP). Clinical trials have shown that *Aimovig*™ significantly reduces the number of migraine episodes. Unfortunately, like most new medications, it is very expensive with a current price of ~$600/monthly injection.

OTHER PAIN MEDICATIONS

Tramadol is a commonly used medication for many types of pain. It is a weak opioid but also has an activity similar to the SNRI antidepressants discussed above. Tramadol is often prescribed for neuropathic pain, as well as some types of non-neuropathic chronic pain, such as low back pain and osteoarthritis. There is less evidence that tramadol is effective in acute pain or post-operative pain.

Tramadol was developed in Germany in the 1970s and approved by the FDA in 1995. It is widely used as an alternative to the strong opioids. Tramadol is a Schedule IV drug, meaning that it is less restricted than other opioids (Table 2). Although it is a weaker drug, it still has some potential for abuse. (43) Moreover, not all individuals will obtain pain relief from Tramadol, since its effectiveness can be determined by an individual's genetic composition (see Chapter 10).

Tapentadol, sold under the brand name *Nycynta*™, is another medication with multiple mechanisms of action that is prescribed for both neuropathic and non-neuropathic pain. Tapentadol acts on opioid receptors, similarly to tramadol, but is more potent and is a Schedule II drug. It also blocks the reuptake of norepinephrine, but not serotonin.

CONCLUSION

Many types of pain-relieving medications are available today, but none of them is ideal. Current pain medications have either limited efficacy and/or unacceptable side effects. This is especially true for medications to relieve neuropathic pain, since they usually provide only a maximum of 30% pain relief at tolerable doses.

The situation is somewhat better for non-neuropathic pain. Existing medications can relieve many types of non-neuropathic pain, but they are not issue-free. The commonly used NSAIDs and acetaminophen (*Tylenol*™) relieve mild pain, but their long-term use can have serious side effects. Currently, the strong opioids are the only oral medications which effectively relieve moderate or severe pain. Unfortunately, the opioids can be easily abused. As discussed in the next chapter, use of opioids for pain relief is controversial and highly debated today.

Because there is a large unmet medical need for pain relief, pharmaceutical companies have been working to identify better drugs to alleviate pain. The "Holy Grail" would be a new drug which has the effectiveness of opioids in relieving pain but does not have abuse potential. Chapter 8 discusses some of the ongoing research to discover and develop better pain medications.

CHAPTER 7

PRESCRIPTION OPIOIDS: EVIL DRUGS OR ESSENTIAL MEDICATIONS FOR PAIN RELIEF?

Opioids have been used for millennia to relieve pain, as discussed in Chapter 6. Although it has been known for a long time that opioids can be readily abused, the problems of opioid abuse have reached epidemic proportions in the US. This chapter discusses some of the causes of the current opioid crisis. Blame for the crisis is multi-factorial. Large pharmaceutical companies which downplayed opioid risks, as well as physicians who over-prescribed these strong medications, certainly have contributed to the problem. These factors are well-known. Less well-known are problems in the generic drug industry and the distribution system, from manufacturers to wholesale distributors and then to pharmacies. However, in spite of the issues associated with opioids, it must be remembered that many patients do receive relief of debilitating pain through legitimate use of prescription opioids. This chapter attempts to provide a balanced assessment of the risks and benefits of prescription opioids for pain relief.

Due to the opioid abuse crisis, the media, regulatory agencies, and various organizations today frequently express the view that opioid use for pain relief must be more effectively controlled and greatly reduced. There is considerable discussion and controversy about which patients, if any, should receive prescription opioids for pain relief. The *long-term* use of opioids to manage chronic pain is especially controversial. Fears of opioid addiction are widespread. Contemporary media, especially television and tabloid newspapers, emphasize the negative aspects of opioids, without pointing out that many people do take prescription opioids responsibly to relieve their pain. This chapter will discuss the results of multiple studies to assess the actual risk of addiction. The chapter will also show that increased regulations and reluctance of physicians to prescribe opioids are limiting the ability of patients to obtain the medications they need for relief of debilitating pain. Finally, this chapter will describe recent efforts to develop formulations of opioids with reduced potential for abuse, as well as current treatments for people who have become addicted.

SHORT-TERM USE OF OPIOIDS TO RELIEVE MODERATE TO SEVERE ACUTE PAIN

Opioids are very effective in relieving acute moderate to severe pain. They are widely prescribed following surgery while a patient is in the hospital and also commonly provided to patients upon release from the hospital or after outpatient surgical procedures. Patients with post-surgical pain are expected to utilize the opioids only until pain subsides as healing occurs. These patients then usually return to their normal activities and exhibit little or no risk for abuse or addiction. Opioids are also the most common drugs for pain relief in terminally ill patients, especially those with cancer. (1)

Certainly, the strong opioids have their limitations and concerns, but there are no other current medications which can relieve severe pain. The World Health Organization (WHO) has provided guidelines for prescribing opioids (see Table 1 in Chapter 6). The WHO has stated that opioids are "absolutely necessary" when pain is moderate to severe. Although these guidelines were originally intended for cancer pain, they are also widely followed to manage severe acute pain associated with a variety of injuries and conditions.

OPIOIDS: IMPORTANT DRUGS FOR ACUTE PAIN, BUT WHAT ABOUT CHRONIC PAIN?

In addition to the short-term use of opioids to relieve acute pain, 5 to 8 million Americans rely on opioids to manage chronic pain. (2) But some physicians today are questioning whether opioids are actually effective in relieving chronic pain. Unfortunately, there is not much well-established guidance. Although excellent reviews have been published recently, none of the studies cited in these reviews have appropriately evaluated the effectiveness of opioids for chronic pain over long periods of time. (3) Health care providers must rely on their clinical judgment, and perhaps personal biases, in deciding whether to prescribe an opioid for a particular chronic pain patient. (2)

Statements in the media can be misleading. For example, the first sentence in an editorial published by the *New York Times* in 2015 stated that a new review has "found no solid evidence that opioids are effective in relieving long-term chronic pain." (4) Although this statement is factually correct, it can easily be misinterpreted. Some might incorrectly conclude that studies have determined that opioids are ineffective for long term relief of chronic pain. But this is *not* what the cited review states. The review actually says "reliable conclusions about the effectiveness of long-term opioid therapy for chronic pain *are not possible* [my italics] due to the paucity of research to date." (3) Considering only studies which had non-opioid comparison groups, the researchers found "no study of opioid therapy...[that] evaluated long-term (>1 year) outcomes related to pain, function, or quality of life." (3) Most of the randomized, placebo-controlled trials lasted less than six weeks and almost all lasted less than sixteen weeks. (3, 5) The *New York Times* editorial did acknowledge that studies cited in the review were all short term, but then stated: "It is extremely reckless to allow opioid usage and deaths to soar in the absence of proof that the treatment is effective." (4) I would argue that it is also extremely reckless to deny patients pain-relieving medications when needed. Clearly, new studies are needed to evaluate the long-term effectiveness of opioids in relieving chronic pain.

One recent study did compare opioid medications with either NSAIDs or acetaminophen for relief of chronic back pain and osteoarthritis pain. This 12-month study of 240 patients found that the opioids did not provide greater pain relief than non-opioid medications. (6) Moreover, the patients taking non-opioid medications had fewer side effects. (6) The logical conclusion was that other medications should be tried first and that opioids should be prescribed only if pain relief was not adequate with other medications. (6)

Certainly, studies such as these are important, but they have limitations. Further research should evaluate large numbers of patients with each type of chronic pain separately, since different pain types may vary in response to a particular medication. In addition, since the pain an individual experiences is due to many factors, patients should ideally be further subdivided according to age, sex, and other categories in order to determine which types of pain patients may receive the most benefit from a given medication.

An independent panel, which was organized by the US National

Institutes of Health (NIH), issued recommendations in 2017 about the use of opioids for chronic pain. In an interview with *Medscape Medical News*, Dr. David Reuben, who was the lead author of the NIH report, stated that is it not currently known which types of pain respond best to opioids and that considerably more research should be devoted to this topic. (7) So, the jury is still out regarding the effectiveness of opioids for chronic pain.

But recently, several physicians have stated that long-term opioid therapy *can* be appropriate for some patients and that it would be an overreaction to deny opioids for chronic pain patients who have not received relief from other treatments. (7-9) Physicians must have the freedom to decide when to prescribe opioids for pain relief. It is also important to remember that none of the current pain-relieving medications is perfect (see Chapter 6). Side effects and/or inadequate pain relief are potential issues with all types of existing analgesics, so options must be available. Excessive regulations and restrictions on one entire class of pain medication, i.e., the opioids, will likely lead to more pain and suffering.

What do patients themselves tell us about their experiences with opioids for relief of chronic pain? The Washington Post Kaiser Family Foundation conducted a poll of people who had used opioids for an extended period of time for pain relief. The poll found that 92% of these patients said that prescription opioids did reduce their pain at least somewhat; 53% said that these medications relieved pain "very well" and 42% said that they "had a positive impact on their physical health." (10) Two-thirds of the patients taking opioids said that the pain relief they obtained was worth the risk and that the medications had greatly improved their lives. Over 80% of these patients said that they had tried non-narcotic medications, but more than half said that they were ineffective. (11)

OPIOID ABUSE

Extent and Causes of the Problem

Although opioids effectively relieve severe acute pain and chronic pain for some individuals, it is well known that opioids have serious issues. Opioid abuse has increased substantially over the past few decades and is a major public health problem. Almost daily, the media report deaths from opioid overdoses. Heart-rending stories relate the tragic experiences of those who have lost a loved one to an opioid-induced death. Clearly, such tragedies must be reduced.

The Centers for Disease Control and Prevention (CDC) reported over 33,000 deaths involving opioids in the US in 2015. (12, 13) These deaths exceeded those from car accidents or guns! But it is important to note that more of these deaths are increasingly due to opioid "street drugs," including heroin and fentanyl, rather than prescription opioids. Not only the absolute number, but also the increase in deaths in 2015 and 2016 were primarily driven by heroin and especially illicitly manufactured fentanyl. (12-19)

Opioid abusers often use heroin because it can be less expensive on the street, easier to adapt for IV administration, more potent, and more readily available than prescription opioids. The retail cost of pure heroin decreased ~6-fold between 1982 and 2012. (20) Not surprisingly, this price drop strongly correlated with an increase in hospitalizations resulting from heroin overdoses. (21)

Fentanyl is an important opioid medication given by IV injection in emergency departments to relieve severe acute pain. But the problem arises when fentanyl is manufactured and imported illicitly. Fentanyl is approximately fifty times more potent than heroin and it is often mixed with heroin or other drugs for sale on the street. Heroin users know what a "safe" dose is for them. However, overdosing can easily occur when individuals think they are injecting only heroin, but instead the drug also contains the much more potent fentanyl. Thus, the usual safe dose becomes an overdose with often fatal results. Overdose deaths in the US from fentanyl increased more than six fold between 2010 and 2016, with the sharpest increase from 2015 to 2016. Illicit synthetic opioids, primarily fentanyl, contributed to 14% of opioid-related overdose deaths in 2010, 29% in 2015, and nearly 50% in 2016. (17-18)

Although heroin and fentanyl are responsible for an increasingly large percentage of overdose deaths, it is the abuse of prescription opioids that gets the most attention. Diversion of legitimately prescribed opioid medications is often the initial event leading to subsequent abuse. The journalist and author Maia Szalavitz pointed out that 75% of heroin addicts under treatment in 2016 began drug use with prescription opioids, but most of these individuals had obtained them illicitly from friends or relatives. (22)

Patients often receive prescriptions for excessive numbers of opioid pills following surgery or other painful medical conditions. Ultimately, many of these pills are not used by the patients themselves. Instead, they end up in unlocked medicine cabinets, where others have ready access. Teenagers are particularly vulnerable to the temptations of drugs, including those readily available due to carelessness of their parents. As with guns, it is imperative to take sufficient precautions by safely storing all medications, especially opioids. Unused prescription opioids can also end up in illegal sales on the street. Reducing the number of pills per prescription and safeguarding medications in the home are commonsense methods to reduce abuse and diversion of prescription opioids.

Several large pharmaceutical companies certainly bear responsibility for contributing to the current opioid abuse crisis by downplaying the risks of these powerful medications (see below). But newly released documents have pointed out that smaller generic companies were actually supplying the majority of prescription opioids by 2006. (23) A database at the Drug Enforcement Agency

(DEA) indicated that one generic company produced more than eighty opioid pills for each person in the US! Problems in the whole-sale distribution system of prescription drugs also contributed to opioid abuse. (24) In some cases, wholesale distributors supplied large amounts of opioids to pain clinics and pharmacies even when illegal activities were suspected. (24) According to data from the DEA and the CDC, published by the *Washington Post*, some regions of the US, e.g., coastal South Carolina, southeastern Colorado, and parts of Arizona had highly excessive amounts of prescription opioids, with greater than 1 gram per each individual living in the region! (24) Currently there is a major effort in the US to reduce diversion of prescription opioids into illegal hands through better enforcement of existing DEA regulations of the drug distribution system.

Although diversion of prescription opioids has often been the start of opioid abuse, heroin has recently become a more com-mon initiating opioid. In 2005, fewer than 10% of people entering a substance abuse treatment program said they started with heroin, whereas by 2015 this had increased to 33%. (25) It is likely that more people turned to heroin as greater controls were placed on prescription opioids and the price of heroin in the street decreased.

How Great Is the Risk of Opioid Addiction for Pain Patients?

So far, we have talked about opioid abuse by people who are using illegal drugs or drugs that had not been prescribed for them. But how prevalent are opioid abuse and addiction among patients who are responsibly taking prescription opioids for pain relief? Does the risk of opioid addiction outweigh the potential benefit of substantial pain relief?

No medication is devoid of risk, but it is the balance between benefits and risks that must be considered. Many people think the risk of opioids is so great that they continue to suffer from unrelieved pain and are unable to live normal lives. Some of my own friends and family have said that they would rather suffer from pain than risk opioid addiction. But contrary to popular opinion and many reports in the media, several analyses have shown that most people who take prescription opioids for pain relief do *not* become addicted or abuse their medications. (3, 22, 26, 27)

Thirty years ago, the noted pain specialist Kathleen Foley cited multiple references supporting the conclusion that "chronic opioid therapy for patients with nonmalignant pain.... is not associated with substance abuse or psychological dependence," *if* there was no previous history of addiction. (26)

In 1980 a small study was published which many people think substantially contributed to the subsequent opioid abuse crisis. (28) The problem isn't with the study itself, but rather with the inappropriate interpretation by authors of multiple later publications. The reported study actually stated that the addiction rate of hospitalized patients who were given opioids to relieve pain was less than 0.1%. (29) Unfortunately, the title of this brief publication was misleading, since it stated: "Addiction rare in patients treated with narcotics." Although the low level of addiction reported in this publication specifically occurred in hospitalized patients with no history of addiction, many subsequent authors incorrectly generalized this result to conclude that the risk of opioid addiction among the general population is very low. It seems likely that the authors of the later publications had read only the misleading title and had not carefully read the report itself. Clearly, it is a gross overstatement to conclude that the overall level of addiction in the general population is the same as in patients with no history of addiction who were given opioids only while hospitalized.

In the past, many pharmaceutical companies heavily advertised new opioid medications without appropriately describing their risks for abuse and addiction. Several lawsuits against some pharmaceutical companies are pending. The lawsuits charge that inappropriate heavy marketing contributed substantially to the current opioid abuse situation. Particularly egregious examples are advertisements from Purdue Pharma in the 1990s touting the value of their new opioid medication called *OxyContin*™. (30) Although *OxyContin*™ was originally promoted to relieve severe cancer pain, Purdue Pharma began in 1998 to extensively promote its use for other conditions such as arthritis and back pain. (30) Advertisements produced by Purdue Pharma consistently downplayed the risks of abuse and addiction.

But how great are the actual risks? Recent estimates of the percentages of pain patients who abuse or become addicted to opioids vary widely. A 2015 review of multiple published studies stated that the prevalence of opioid abuse among pain patients who received prescriptions from primary health care providers ranged from 0.6% to 8%, whereas abuse among patients who received opioid medications from pain clinics ranged from 8-16%. (3) However, these were uncontrolled studies of varying quality.

More accurate numbers can be obtained by statistical analysis of combined data from multiple studies. As Maia Szalavitz wrote in the *Washington Post,* "A 2010 Cochrane review – considered the gold standard for basing medical practice on evidence – found an addiction rate of less than 1%" among pain patients who received opioid prescriptions. (22) Specifically, this review found that signs of addiction were reported in only 0.27% of the patients and concluded that long-term pain relief can be achieved in some well-selected patients with a very small risk of abuse or addiction. (27)

Another review, which combined data from all available high-quality studies, calculated a rate of 3.27% for abuse or addiction among chronic non-cancer pain patients. (31) But importantly, this rate decreased substantially to 0.19%, when the assessment included only patients with no previous history of abuse or addiction. (31)

Similarly, another study found that the primary predictors of opioid abuse in pain patients were previous abuse of alcohol or cocaine, or an earlier drug or DUI conviction. There was no correlation between drug abuse and other parameters such as income, education, race, disability, depression, or literacy. (32)

The multiple studies described above clearly show that opioids do carry some risk of addiction. However, the risk of pain patients becoming addicted to prescription opioids, especially in the absence of drug or alcohol abuse, is much lower than the media suggest.

Drug Abuse, Dependence, or Addiction?

The terms drug abuse, dependence, and addiction are often used interchangeably and inappropriately, although the three conditions are quite different. It is important to distinguish among these terms, since misunderstandings can arise from inappropriate usage.

A person who abuses drugs is not necessarily addicted. Abuse can simply mean that a person is taking more pills or taking them more often than prescribed. Taking a drug that has been prescribed to someone else, and of course using street drugs, are also forms of abuse.

The term drug dependence is commonly used interchangeably with addiction, but these two conditions are not the same. Drug dependence means that the individual requires continued use of the drug to prevent the withdrawal symptoms which occur if the medication is not present in the body. The physiology of the person has changed, such that the patient requires the drug to feel normal. Withdrawal symptoms due to physiological dependence are extremely unpleasant.

People with physiological dependence on opioids often live normal productive lives, maintaining careers, family relationships, and social interactions. In contrast, true addiction destroys lives and families. Addiction is sometimes referred to as *psychological* dependence, which occurs in addition to *physiological* dependence. The biological basis for psychological dependence, i.e., true addiction, is not well understood. Those who are addicted become totally preoccupied with obtaining the drug and demonstrate no self-control over its attainment and use, in spite of the many hazards.

Unfortunately, media usually do not distinguish between dependence and actual addiction. The headline in a *Washington Post* article exclaimed: "One-third of long-term users say they are hooked on prescription opioids." (11) The article goes on to state that these individuals say they "became addicted to, or physically dependent," without differentiating between the two. (11) It is addiction that is the public health problem, not dependence. But addiction is much more than a public health problem. Addiction is a disease, *not* a moral failure.

Role of Genetics in Addiction?

There are many factors which determine whether a particular individual may become addicted. One factor may be inherited genetic tendencies. Many laboratory studies have explored the biological and experiential bases of addiction using specific strains of rats and mice. (33) Because each rodent strain is inbred, all animals in a particular strain possess the same basic genetic composition. As such, they are widely used in medical research to study the role of genetics in many diseases or behaviors.

In his book *The Painful Truth*, pain specialist Lynn Webster described studies using different strains of rats which exhibit different tendencies to develop addiction. (34) As he wrote, "One breed — named Fischer 344 – is resistant to addiction. Even after a Fischer rat has been repeatedly injected with a highly addictive substance, the rat will refuse to self-administer the drug when given that option. A second breed – Lewis rats – acts in just the opposite way. They are so genetically predisposed to addiction that, even if the drug they have been given is only slightly addictive, they will do anything to access the drug, even walk across a burning-hot plate to get to it. Then there is a third breed, known as Sprague Dawley rats, whose behavior falls between those of the other two breeds. If subjected to stresses, such as loud music or sleep deprivation, the Sprague Dawley rats will act like Lewis rats and seek the rewards of addictive drugs. If not stressed, they will act like Fischer 344 rats, showing no interest in the drugs." (34) These studies suggest that both genetic and environmental factors contribute to addiction.

Webster goes on to suggest that if similar genetic components to addiction exist in humans, some people will be at higher risk for addiction, like the Lewis rats. A genetically predisposed person may easily become addicted upon chronic opioid use. A small percentage of people may be resistant to addiction, much like the Fischer rats. Webster proposes that the majority of humans may be more like the Sprague Dawley rats, who have low genetic predisposition to addiction, but may become addicted to drugs as a result of circumstances in their lives such as ongoing stress. (34)

The potential role of genetics in human drug addiction or dependence is an ongoing area of research. Several studies have concluded that heritability does contribute to opioid addiction, nicotine and alcohol dependence, as well as cannabis and cocaine use disorders. (35) However, recent attempts to identify specific genes that influence human opioid addiction have not yielded consistent results. (35)

BALANCING PAIN-RELIEVING BENEFITS *VS* RISKS OF PRESCRIPTION OPIOIDS

As discussed in Chapter 5, the importance of pain relief is currently being devalued, due primarily to the opioid abuse crisis. The previous emphasis on the importance of balancing the pain-relieving benefits of opioids vs their risks has diminished. A backlash to the legitimate prescribing of opioids has occurred. Various governmental agencies, as well as the media and advocacy groups, have supported stronger regulations to decrease the prescribing of opioids. The argument is that when fewer opioids are prescribed, there will be less abuse. In theory, this sounds reasonable, but it does not take into account that many pain patients will suffer needlessly if they are not able to obtain their medications. Moreover, when legitimate prescription opioids are unavailable, the black market for unregulated drugs increases. Yes, prescription opioids carry risks, but less so than the uncontrolled drugs with variable potency and purity that are readily available on street corners and back alleys throughout the US.

Increasing Restrictions in the United States

Although the strong opioids, such as hydrocodone, oxycodone, and morphine are the only medications which can provide relief for many patients with moderate or severe pain, barriers to their availability are increasing. The greatest barriers in the US are the increased regulations by governmental agencies and the new restrictions by insurance companies and pharmacies.

In recent years, the Drug Enforcement Agency has established multiple new regulations in an attempt to reduce opioid abuse. One regulation, which took effect mid-2014, limits a prescription for an opioid to a maximum of thirty days' treatment. As a result, a patient taking an opioid long-term to relieve chronic pain has to visit both the doctor's office to obtain the prescription and then the pharmacy with much greater frequency. Such limitations are particularly a problem for the poor, the elderly, and the disabled, who often do not have readily available transportation and must rely on others for their frequent visits to the physician's office and the pharmacy. Many veterans have been taking opioid medications since returning from war and rely upon these medications for pain relief. It is difficult for veterans to obtain these required appointments every thirty days since the US Veteran's Administration (VA) often has long backlogs in available appointments. Also, many veterans live a long distance from the VA hospitals or clinics, complicating their ability to obtain needed medications. (36)

In 2016, the US Centers for Disease Control and Prevention (CDC) published guidelines for prescribing opioids to relieve chronic pain. (37) The document stated that the purpose of these guidelines was to "improve communication between clinicians and patients about the risks and benefit of opioid therapy for chronic pain, improve the safety and effectiveness of pain treatment, and reduce the risks associated with long-term therapy, including opioid use disorder." (37) The guidelines included recommendations regarding the type of opioid prescribed and defined specific maximum doses. Although the CDC stated that these recommendations were only guidelines, some physicians expressed concern that regulatory agencies, insurers, and prescription benefit managers would view the guidelines as providing authorization to limit access to prescription opioids. (38) Also, many health care providers do not have adequate training on pain management, including the use of opioids, and may simply take the guidelines as the final word.

The CDC guidelines caused an immediate reaction from many health care providers. (39) Compounding the concerns was the statement by the Director of the CDC, as quoted in the *Washington Post*, "Opioids carry substantial risks but only uncertain benefits. The risks will outweigh the benefits for the vast majority of patients." (40) A *Medscape* article quoted many physicians who were concerned about the new CDC guidelines. The article ended with this quote from a registered nurse: "CDC, take my pain for a month; you would be on the streets trying to get your next fix. Let the doctors be doctors." (39) Somewhat later, a family practitioner wrote: "I have treated many patients over the last 10-12 years with chronic opiates. The majority seem to be helped with this therapy. Many would lead a life of despair without these meds....As long as they show no signs of impairment, or drug-seeking behaviour, why stop an effective treatment?" (41)

In March 2019, the *New York Times* reported that a letter, signed by over 300 medical experts including former White House drug czars, was being sent to the CDC. (42) This letter expressed concerns that chronic pain patients were being harmed by these guidelines and described multiple patients who had been taking high doses of an opioid for a long time without becoming addicted. (42) The authors of the letter further noted that, as previously feared, the guidelines were being used both by insurers to deny reimbursements and by doctors to stop treating chronic pain patients with opioids. (42) The letter stated: "It is imperative that health care professionals and administrators realize that the guideline does not endorse mandated involuntary dose reduction or discontinuation." (42) *The New York Times* article further quoted an American Medical Association resolution which stated strong objections to the "misapplication" of the guidelines "by pharmacists, health insurers, pharmacy benefit managers, legislatures, and governmental and private regulatory bodies in ways that prevent or limit access to opioid analgesia." (42)

Dr. Kenneth Lin, a family physician at the Georgetown University Medical Center in Washington DC, published a commentary in which he described that he had recently obtained many new patients who had been taking high doses of opioids for years, but now their previous physicians were limiting doses to only those in the CDC guidelines or were no longer prescribing opioids at all. (9) Dr. Lin also pointed out that pharmacies were often refusing to fill the prescriptions due to the CDC guidelines and/or adding additional administrative requirements. (9)

Pharmacy benefit managers have also imposed greater restrictions. Starting in 2017, Express Scripts, which is the largest pharmacy benefits manager in the US, limited the initial opioid prescription to a maximum of seven days, whether the treatment was for acute or chronic pain. Moreover, the default was to dispense the short-acting opioids. Physicians must obtain prior authorization for the long-acting opioids, which often provide better overall pain relief. This prior authorization places an additional administrative burden on physicians and can delay the patient's receipt of the medications. (43) Moreover, some insurance companies have limited the maximum daily dose of opioids and the types of opioids they will cover, citing the CDC guidelines. (42)

Dr. Charles Argoff, a Professor of Neurology at Albany Medical College and Director of the Comprehensive Pain Center at Albany Medical Center in Albany NY, published a commentary expressing his concerns that policymakers are conflating the potential of opioid abuse with use of opioids for pain relief. (44) Dr. Argoff stated that "the concept of undo [sic] harm to people in pain is becoming the new standard of care due to the sudden cessation of treatment that had previously been efficacious. This is clinically unacceptable." (44) He further stated: "The reality is that for millions of people with chronic pain, opioid therapy is effective and safe in helping them to live more comfortable and productive lives." (44)

The current call for more regulations controlling opioid prescriptions has shifted the balance away from the needs of pain patients. It can be legitimately argued that the balance in the past was strongly tilted in the other direction; i.e., towards too much opioid prescribing. The argument is that the earlier increased emphasis on pain relief put pressure on clinicians to prescribe opioids, resulting in large increases in opioid prescriptions. Unfortunately, this increase was associated with more abuse and an increase in deaths from opioid overdoses. Now the pendulum has swung sharply in the other direction, away from aggressive use of opioids for pain relief to severe restrictions on the only medications which can effectively relieve severe pain. Return to a more balanced approach is needed.

"Opiophobia"

Many physicians today are afraid to prescribe opioids for their pain patients. The opioid-prescribing practices of primary care physicians and specialists in pain management are being heavily scrutinized. Certainly, as widely reported in the media, there are some "pill-pushing" doctors who dispense inordinate amounts of opioids, sometimes without even examining the so-called patients. But most physicians who prescribe opioids for their pain patients do so in a compassionate and responsible manner. Health care providers have stated that opioid medications have enabled a much higher quality of life for some pain patients, even including return to work. (45) Nevertheless, there is a growing number of physicians who will only prescribe strong opioids very reluctantly, and many will not prescribe them at all.

One reason for the reluctance to prescribe opioids is concern about attracting the attention of the DEA. In his book *The Painful Truth*, Dr. Lynn Webster describes his encounter with the DEA. (34) In 2010, the DEA barged into his pain clinic and demanded medical records of some of his patients. Clearly the DEA was investigating whether he was inappropriately prescribing opioids. After being under a cloud of suspicion for four years, no further legal action was taken against Webster, but the anguish he suffered was immense.

A similar situation occurred at the office of a nurse practitioner who ran a family medicine clinic. She treated chronic pain patients, but also provided care for other types of patients. However, it was the ~20% of her practice which involved pain management that resulted in a "visit" from the DEA. As at the Webster clinic, the DEA barged into her clinic, but this time the DEA officers were more aggressive. Reportedly at gunpoint, the officers ordered the nurse practitioner, her office staff as well as patients in the waiting room to lie down on the floor with hands behind their backs. The officers confiscated the computers containing all patient records. Without her computers, this health care provider could not send out bills or access information about prior visits of her patients. The accusations against her, combined with a variety of complicating issues, resulted in a long legal struggle. Eventually she was able to preserve her medical license and ability to operate her clinic. (46)

Beside the reluctance of physicians to prescribe opioids, pharmacists may be reluctant to fill opioid prescriptions. Both physicians and pharmacists fear criminal prosecution for prescribing and dispensing opioids. (47) In 2017, the US Department of Justice announced that it will gather data on opioid prescribing and dispensing practices of physicians and pharmacists and will utilize this data to identify those who appear to be contributing to the opioid crisis. (47)

An extreme case of misuse of databases which track opioid prescribing was recently described. The Medical Board of California looked at the correlation between opioid prescribing by physicians and the patients who later overdosed. The board launched investigations into prescribing practices of over 400 physicians and, as of January 2019, at least twenty-three physicians had been formally accused of negligence and excessive prescribing. Many physicians responded by calling this probe a "witch hunt." (48)

In addition to the fear of being investigated by government agencies, many physicians and pharmacists themselves are concerned that opioid misuse by one of their patients will result in an overdose and that the patient's family and friends will consider them responsible. Between 40 and 50% of physicians and pharmacists surveyed said that they feared being sued for liability in the case of an opioid overdose death. (47) Moreover, half of physicians and 62% of pharmacists expressed fear that they might become the victim of violence if they refused to write or fill an opioid prescription for a patient. (47) Yes, there are safeguards that health care providers can incorporate into their practices when prescribing opioids. But the added administrative burden can be overwhelming for busy practices, lapses in procedures can occur, and some patients indeed may misuse their prescribed opioids.

Due to concerns about prescribing opioids and increased regulations, prescription rates for opioids decreased each year from 2013 to 2016. (49, 50) The decrease, which was observed in 49 states, was the first sustained decrease in opioid prescriptions since 1996. (50) A new report from Reuters Health has found that physicians decreased the number of new opioid prescriptions they wrote by more than 50% between 2012 and 2017. (51)

Impact of "Opiophobia" on Pain Patients

The widespread fear of opioids is a major cause of inadequate pain relief today. The increased regulations on prescribing opioids are causing more pain and suffering. Judith A. Paice, Research Professor at the Robert H. Lurie Comprehensive Cancer Center of Northwestern University, Chicago, has stated that "the problem [of inadequate pain relief] in the United States may be worsening through the unintentional consequences associated with measures to limit the opioid abuse epidemic." (52)

In 2016, the Washington Post Kaiser Family Foundation asked patients with various types of chronic pain about their experience with obtaining prescription opioids. The survey found that "two-thirds of long-term users said that they are concerned that efforts to decrease abuse of prescription painkillers could make it more difficult to obtain them. Nearly 6 in 10 say that as it is [in 2016], prescription painkillers are difficult to obtain for medical purposes." (10) By 2018 the situation had gotten worse, as more regulations were instituted. Even cancer patients and survivors reported great-er difficulty in obtaining prescription opioids in May 2018 compared with late 2016, according to a survey conducted by the American Cancer Society. (53) Issues identified in this survey included: not being able to get an opioid because a physician would not prescribe the medication; a pharmacy did not have it in stock; the pharmacist would not fill the prescription even if the opioid was in stock; the pharmacist questioned the patient why he needed the medication; insurance no longer covered the opioid; dispensing was restricted to a single pharmacy; and reduction in the number of pills per pre-scription. (53)

A "Perspective" published in 2018 in the *New England Journal of Medicine* described a patient who had multiple injuries from a motorcycle accident and then developed chronic pain. (54) This pa-tient had been taking oxycodone and other pain-relieving medica-tions for two years and all follow-up visits to the doctor showed that he was closely adhering to his medication regimen. But sub-sequently, his doctor told him that she would no longer prescribe oxycodone. He then went to six other doctors who also refused to prescribe oxycodone. In desperation he went to a pain clinic, tear-fully explaining that he was afraid he would need to instead buy opioids on the street. Mercifully, the pain clinic entered him into a multidisciplinary pain program which would provide opioids when needed. The pain clinic said that this was not an isolated case, since they had seen numerous patients like this. (54)

In 2018, 40% of primary care clinics in Michigan stated that their health care providers would *not* accept new patients who were cur-rently taking prescription opioids for pain relief. (55) The authors of this report pointed out that there could be unintended conse-quences of reduced primary care access to prescription opioids, in-cluding greater use of illicit drugs. (55) Indeed, some chronic pain patients do use illicit drugs. (56) Due to the difficulty in obtaining effective pain medications from their physicians, more chronic pain patients may turn to illicit drugs.

The Criminalization Model and the War on Drugs

A report from the Opioid Policy Initiative has stated that regulations regarding opioid prescribing and availability in Europe are more consistent with a " 'criminalization model' to mitigate crime and addiction rather than a 'public health model' to facilitate care and reduce harms." (57) This type of "criminalization model" has been pervasive in the US for decades.

President Nixon declared a "war on drugs" in 1971 in response to drug use by veterans returning from the Vietnam War and to increased drug use among the overall population. The Nixon administration increased the size of federal drug control agencies and instituted policies such as mandatory sentencing for drug violations. The Rockefeller Drug Laws, which were established in 1973 in New York, became the basis for criminalization of drug use in the US. Very large amounts of money have been spent by federal, state and local governments in the war on drugs over the past ~50 years, yet drug use and abuse in the US have not decreased, but instead have increased. It is important to remember that we are not at war with those who are addicted to opioids. Drug abuse is a public health problem. Increased access to treatment, rather than increased incarceration, is needed. The "war on drugs" terminology also carries a broader undercurrent of perceived criminality. Patients often feel they are being treated like criminals when they request opioids to relieve their pain.

I suggest that the criminalization model and the war on drugs are significantly present in the current climate of opiophobia with frequently tragic results. Increased regulations are causing more people to turn to illicit drugs readily available on the streets of cities, suburbs, small towns, and rural areas. Even though the number of opioid prescriptions has decreased (49, 50), the deaths from opioid overdoses continue to rise. (14) Is it simply too soon for the decrease in opioid prescriptions to be reflected in a reduction of overdoses? Alternatively, as legitimate opioid prescriptions decrease, are more people turning to illegal drugs? The New York City borough of Staten Island has reported that the restrictions on opioid prescribing have caused some pain patients to turn to heroin obtained on the street. (58) Indeed, as discussed earlier in this chapter, heroin and illicit fentanyl are responsible for much of the recent increase in deaths from opioid overdoses.

Haven't we learned lessons from history? Attempts to correct social problems through restrictive laws often fail or have unintended consequences. One prominent example is the 18th amendment to the US Constitution. This amendment, which was ratified as part of the Constitution in 1919, mandated a nationwide ban on all aspects of production and sale of alcoholic beverages. The amendment was the result of a reform movement led by Protestants in rural areas and by social progressives in both the Democratic and Republican parties. Several types of social problems were becoming rampant in many urban areas, not only in the US but also in Europe. Reform movements grew, especially in England and the US. The reform movement in the US succeeded in spreading its conviction that the root of social ills was "devil rum" and all other alcoholic beverages. As a result, the 18th amendment to the US Constitution was adopted and then implemented in 1920 through passage of the Volstead Act.

However, this attempt to abolish social ills through highly restrictive laws concerning production and sale of alcohol was a failure! In spite of the ban, alcoholic beverages were widely available during the Prohibition Era if one knew where to find them. Speakeasy clubs and other underground sources of alcoholic beverages emerged and gained a considerable foothold. An unintended consequence of the

18th amendment was the growth of organized crime in the 1920s. Organized crime provided a source of the banned alcohol. Horrific gang-related crimes increased during the 1920s. Eventually it became apparent that the ban on alcoholic beverages did not provide the solution to societal ills! The 21st Amendment to the US Constitution, which repealed the 18th amendment, was ratified in 1933.

As during the Prohibition Era, when individuals found ways to obtain banned alcoholic beverages and criminal activities expanded, I suggest that a similar situation exists today regarding opioids. As laws have become more restrictive for legal opioid medications, criminal activities have expanded. Heroin and other dangerous illegal drugs are readily available on street corners, alleys, and byways in urban, suburban, and rural areas of the US. When alcohol or prescription opioids are not available for legitimate use, people will find alternative sources. It seems unlikely that a society free of the dangers of opioids, alcohol, and other agents susceptible to abuse can ever be achieved simply through increased governmental regulations.

Unfortunately, the extreme rhetoric often used in the United States due to the opioid crisis is beginning to spread throughout the world. Meg O'Brien, the founder of Treat the Pain, an advocacy organization dedicated to relieving pain in poor countries, described this concern in a recent article in the *New York ScienceTimes*. She stated that the American delegation to the United Nations' International Narcotics Control Board "uses frightening war-on-drugs rhetoric….that has a chilling effect on developing countries…. But it's ridiculous – the U.S. also has an obesity epidemic, but no one is proposing that we withhold food aid from South Sudan." (59)

The Global Opioid Policy Initiative (GOPI) evaluated the availability of opioids, specifically for cancer pain. (57) One of the authors of the GOPI report, Dr. Nathan Cherny, stated that there is "a pandemic of over-regulation in much of the developing world that is making it catastrophically difficult to provide basic medication to relieve strong cancer pain." (60) Stringent governmental regulations have limited opioid availability. (61) In some sub-Saharan African countries, patients must register with local police departments to obtain morphine and often must travel many miles under difficult conditions to obtain pain relief. (60)

ABUSE-DETERRENT OPIOID PRODUCTS

Although most health care providers acknowledge that opioids are important medications to relieve severe pain and should be available for patients who need them, the risks of prescription opioid abuse can't be ignored. Certainly the pharmaceutical industry is not blameless in the rise of prescription opioid abuse, but I would point out that the industry has explored several ways to develop new opioid products which retain the ability to relieve moderate and severe pain, but are less likely to be abused.

New Formulations

One approach to reduce abuse potential is to modify the formulation in the pill containing an opioid. One of the earliest drugs with this approach *was Oxycontin*™ (oxycodone) developed by Purdue Pharma in 1995. This formulation was designed to release the oxycodone more slowly and therefore prevent the rapid generation of high concentrations that cause euphoria. However, *Oxycontin*™ had only limited ability to reduce abuse since it was quickly discovered that crushing an *OxyContin*™ tablet generated a powder which could be inhaled. Inhalation of the powder overcame the time-release properties and restored the rapid euphoria. Such was the origin of the wide-spread abuse of *OxyContin*™ in the US.

Several other formulations have been developed more recently. Some of these formulations aim to reduce abuse by making it more difficult for the opioid to be injected, which is one of the primary methods for abuse. Zogenix Inc has developed a formulation of the opioid hydrocodone, based on their proprietary *BeadTek* technology. The company has stated that this technology "incorporates well-known pharmaceutical excipients that immediately form a viscous gel when crushed and dissolved in liquids or solvents," thereby making it more difficult to solubilize the hydrocodone for injection. (62) This product, known as *Zohydro* ER, was approved by the FDA in 2015 "for chronic pain which is severe enough to require daily around-the-clock, long-term opioid treatment." (62, 63)

Another proprietary new technology called Guardian has been developed by the Egalet Corporation. This technology applies the well-known manufacturing injection molding process to produce hard tablets that are highly resistant to a variety of physical manipulation methods. The hard tablets are difficult to crush and form a viscous gel if the contents are dissolved. An abuse-deterrent formulation of morphine, known as *Arymo ER*™, was developed using this technology. *Arymo ER*™ was approved by the FDA in 2017. The Egalet Corporation has stated that it is nearly impossible to extract morphine from these tablets so that it can be injected, which is the primary route for abuse of morphine. (64, 65)

The Egalet Corporation also has developed a new abuse-deterrent form of oxycodone using the Guardian Technology. According to Egalet, this technology makes it extremely difficult to get the oxycodone into a power form for "snorting," which is a major route for abuse of oxycodone. The Egalet Corporation issued a press release in 2017 stating that their oxycodone tablet (currently known as Egalet-002) effectively relieved moderate-to-severe chronic low back pain in late stage clinical trials. (66) However, at the time of submitting this book for publication, Egalet-002 had not yet entered the marketplace.

Addition of an Antagonist

Another approach to reducing abuse of opioids combines morphine or oxycodone with a substance known as an opioid antagonist. To understand this approach, it is necessary to present some basic pharmacology on how drugs act. In general, drugs act by binding to specific sites on defined proteins, which are either enzymes or receptors. After drugs such as morphine or oxycodone bind to specific cell-surface receptors, they initiate a series of events inside the cell. These opioids and other drugs which elicit a cellular response are called "agonists." In contrast, other drugs, which block the effects of agonists, are called "antagonists."

The idea behind this approach is that the antagonist would block the euphoria, while the agonist would provide pain relief. However, it is currently thought that one type of opioid receptor, known as the μ receptor, is the primary receptor involved in both relieving pain and generating the euphoria. Since opioid agonists and antagonists likely compete for binding to the same receptors, how can the antagonist block the euphoria but still allow full pain relief?

One approach is to separate the agonist and antagonist into different compartments of a capsule. The concept is that when an intact pill is swallowed, only the agonist would be released from its compartment, allowing full pain-relieving effects of morphine or other opioid agonists. However, if the pill is crushed to enable inhalation or injection, the antagonist in the other compartment would also be released. Pfizer has developed a combination of morphine with the antagonist naltrexone using this technology. This drug is marketed under the name *EMBEDA*®. The FDA has approved an updated label for *EMBEDA*® stating that it has "properties that are expected to reduce abuse via the oral and intranasal (snorting) routes when crushed." (67) Importantly, *EMBEDA*® has been reported to retain the full pain-relieving properties of morphine, demonstrating that when the capsules are taken orally, this technology successfully keeps the antagonist sequestered. (68) This physical separation of the agonist from the antagonist holds promise in reducing abuse of prescription opioids. However, *EMBEDA®* may still have potential for abuse and it is expensive, currently costing around $200 for 30 capsules.

It remains to be seen whether these new formulations of prescription opioids and/or the combinations of an opioid agonist with an antagonist will have a significant impact on the overall problem of opioid abuse. A 2018 review concluded that it is too soon to say whether these new abuse-deterrent methods have "altered the trajectory of opioid overdose and addiction," but post-marketing studies of the FDA approved products are ongoing and other products are still in development. (69)

URGENT NEED TO EXPAND TREATMENT FOR THOSE ADDICTED TO OPIOIDS

This chapter has discussed efforts to reduce abuse of prescription opioids, including increased regulations and new products with lower potential for abuse and addiction. But we must not lose sight of the fact that many people today are addicted not to prescription opioids, but rather to heroin and other street drugs. Unfortunately, many people believe that drug addiction is a moral failure, which can be overcome simply through abstinence and will power. This belief overlooks the biological basis for addiction and results in unnecessary suffering and loss of human life. *Addiction is a disease, not a moral failing.* Nevertheless, the stigma associated with addiction prevents many individuals from obtaining the help they need. One recent estimate is that only 10% of people in the US with opioid abuse problems actually receive treatment. (70)

Opioid abuse and addiction often accompany despair and mental illness. Patrick J. Kennedy, a former Representative in the US Congress and son of the late Senator Ted Kennedy, was previously addicted to opioid pain killers. In an article published by the *Washington Post*, Kennedy advocated for considering opioid addiction under the overall umbrella of mental illness. (71) As he stated, "We will not be able to address this new and troubling addiction issue until we embrace the idea that all addiction care, and all mental health care, needs to be delivered in a radically different, holistic way – fully integrated into the rest of our medical care, and no longer viewed, as it has been too often, as palliative care for moral failings or 'demons'." (71)

Governmental Initiatives to Address Opioid Addiction

City, state, and federal government agencies and lawmakers in the US have begun to address opioid abuse as a public health crisis. In 2016, I attended a Roundtable entitled *America's Insatiable Demand for Drugs: Examining Alternative Approaches*, which was organized by the US Senate Committee on Homeland Security and Governmental Affairs. (72) The session included panelists with differing opinions about these approaches.

One of the panelists was Frederick Ryan, Chief of Police in Arlington, Massachusetts. Ryan, who has thirty years of experience in the police force, also heads a drug addiction treatment program in which police are directing drug addicts to treatment, rather than arresting them. Ryan emphasized that addiction is a disease and does not warrant incarceration. As he said, we are not at war with drug addicts. He also stated that the threat of arrest does not deter drug addicts from further drug use. (72)

Another witness was D. Scott MacDonald from the Providence Crosstown Clinic in Vancouver, Canada. He described two clinics in Vancouver that manage the long-term treatment of drug addicts through a program of supervised opioid injections. These are not "methadone clinics" (see below) but rather they are clinics which provide patients with morphine or other prescription opioids that they would have otherwise obtained illegally on the street. Dr. MacDonald stated that because these patients receive opioids from the clinic, they are less likely to contribute to the societal ills that often accompany drug addiction. (72) Similarly, another panelist Ethan Nadelmann, who is the founder of the Drug Policy Alliance which promotes alternative approaches to the "failed war on drugs," pointed out that supervised provision of prescription opioids, which started in Switzerland, has also been successfully used in other countries. (72) Dr. Nadelmann said that sixty-six cities in nine countries had safe supervised injection facilities in 2016, similar to the ones described by Dr. MacDonald. He went on to say that twenty years of experience with this approach in Europe has led to a decrease in drug-related crime and has enabled many people to return to a functional role in society and to hold productive jobs. (72)

Taking the opposite point of view on supervised injection sites was David W. Murray from the Hudson Institute, which is a public policy think tank in Washington DC. He stated that he is totally opposed to controlled injection sites for drug addicts and quoted others who said that claims of their effectiveness are overstated. His opinion was that it would be wrong for the US government to legalize and encourage such an approach. (72)

Interestingly, a century ago some cities in the United States did have clinics which provided addicts with legal drugs to prevent them from turning to illicit drugs and accompanying crime. (28, 73) However by 1923, the US federal government had essentially shut down all these clinics. (28, 73) As a recent *New York Times* editorial stated, the shutdown decision was based on the view that "it was wrong to keep supplying drugs to people who had become dependent on them – a view that is, regrettably, still widespread today." (28)

In January 2018, *Morning Edition* on National Public Radio reported that officials in Philadelphia had proposed opening a medically supervised injection site for people suffering from opioid addiction. (74) The new district attorney of Philadelphia stated that users of opioids would not be prosecuted at such a safe injection site. But as expected, there was much resistance, not only from local officials and residents, but also from the federal government. Several other US cities have also considered establishing safe injection sites (74, 75), although none exist at the time of writing this chapter.

CURRENT TREATMENTS FOR OPIOID ADDICTION

Fortunately, other less controversial approaches to the problem of opioid addiction currently do exist in the US. For example, programs similar to Alcoholics Anonymous help patients overcome drug addiction. Most of these programs utilize an approach based on total abstinence from all opioid-type drugs. Following a period of detoxification, patients enter a residential program focused on counseling and group therapy. Although many patients previously addicted to opioids do graduate from the program drug-free, relapse rates are high. A significant percent does not remain drug-free for the long-term and instead returns to the use of opioids. A person who had been in an abstinence-only program and then relapses has a very high risk of a fatal overdose, since the person's tolerance for opioids has substantially decreased. (76)

Addiction is much more than a behavioral problem, since it also has a major physiological component. The brain of an addicted person has changed, and addiction can be considered a *bona fide* disease. As with other diseases, addiction can be treated with medications rather than by abstinence alone.

An example of this approach is the well-known methadone program, which was established in the 1960s and is still in use today. When appropriately utilized, a single dose of methadone prevents withdrawal effects and reduces drug cravings for ~24 hours without causing sedation or euphoria. Methadone treatment has had considerable long-term success in keeping people from resorting to illicit drugs. However, methadone can be administered by only a few clinics and most patients must go to the clinic every day to obtain the medication. (76) Due to the ongoing problems of opioid addiction, more methadone clinics have opened in the past 2-4 years. Originally, these clinics were primarily in major cities, but recently there has been some expansion also into rural and suburban areas. (77) Unfortunately, the temptation to get "high" by using heroin or other readily available street drugs, instead of going to the methadone clinic, is often too great.

A promising new development to treat drug addiction utilizes a different drug, called buprenorphine. Like methadone, the opioid buprenorphine reduces cravings, blocks withdrawal, and does not cause euphoria or sedation. But buprenorphine has a somewhat different mechanism of action. (76)

In the US, an addiction treatment center in Oregon, known as Beyond Addictions, began to utilize buprenorphine in 2007 to relieve cravings for opioids. Dr. Marvin Seppala, who established the Beyond Addictions program, observed that patients who received buprenorphine did not relapse or overdose as often as patients who were treated using only the abstinence/counseling approach. (76)

Subsequently, extensive scientific reviews and several agencies and organizations, including the US Institute of Medicine, the US National Institute on Drug Abuse and the WHO, have confirmed that treatment with medications combined with counseling is substantially more effective than the abstinence/counseling approach in treating opioid addiction. (76-79) An article in the *Washington Post* stated: "The research is unassailable. Staying in recovery and avoiding relapse for at least a year is more than twice as likely with medications as without them." (76) Another article in the

Washington Post cited a British study which found that people who received medication-based maintenance treatment had half the death rate of those who were in programs that required total abstinence. (24) France has reportedly reduced overdoses from heroin by ~80% since buprenorphine became readily available beginning in 1995. (28) Some physicians have pointed out that buprenorphine has enabled patients to return to a more active role in society, since buprenorphine does not cause the sedation associated with morphine, oxycodone, or other opioids.

However, resistance to using medications to treat opioid addiction continues to be very strong among many people, insurance companies, and governmental agencies. Some physicians, psychiatrists, psychologists, social workers, and members of the general population regard medication-based treatment as simply trading one addiction for another, without acknowledging that medication-based treatment can be life-saving.

Only a small percentage of people addicted to opioids receive medication-based treatment today. (76-78) Although the number of methadone clinics has expanded recently, they are still inadequate. In theory, it should be easier for a patient to receive buprenorphine than methadone to manage addiction. Primary care clinicians, in addition to pain and addiction specialists, can prescribe buprenorphine after obtaining specific credentials. The prescription can then be filled at a pharmacy and taken home for daily oral administration. (77, 79) In 2018, the American Medical Association reported that there was a 42% increase in the number of physicians licensed to prescribe buprenorphine over the previous year. (80). Nevertheless, it appears that fewer than 5% of eligible clinicians had this license in 2018. (77) Moreover, each credentialed health care provider is limited in the number of patients he can treat with buprenorphine, although this number has recently increased. (79) Hopefully in the future, many more patients will be able to receive a prescription for buprenorphine from their primary care physician's office rather than needing to go to a specialized methadone clinic. Importantly, a few hospitals in the US are beginning to offer buprenorphine treatment in their emergency rooms for opioid overdose victims. (81) Such proactive efforts may encourage these patients to pursue ongoing treatment for addiction.

A new device containing buprenorphine was approved by the FDA in 2016. This device, known as *Probuphine*™, consists of four little rods that are implanted under the skin on the inside of the upper arm and delivers a constant low-level dose of buprenorphine for as long as six months. (82) The continued low dose of buprenorphine is expected to substantially reduce opioid craving and reversion to illicit drugs. (82) Since the implanted device lasts for several months, compliance issues are greatly reduced. Also, it is expected that *Probuphine*™ would not have the diversion issues that can occur with oral buprenorphine.

Another approach to treating addiction is use of the opioid *antagonist* naltrexone, rather than an opioid agonist such as buprenorphine or methadone (see discussion earlier in this chapter about agonists and antagonists). Naltrexone is expected to prevent, or at least reduce, the use of opioid street drugs, since it blocks the opioid-induced "high." Because naltrexone is not a narcotic, it is easily prescribed by physicians and overcomes much of the reluctance to use methadone and buprenorphine to treat opioid addiction. An injectable form of extended-release naltrexone has been approved by the FDA and is currently marketed as the drug *Vivitrol*™. (83) Only one dose a month is needed. However, because it blocks the action of opioids, patients must go through a painful detoxification period before they can begin using *Vivitrol*™. Severe withdrawal symptoms occur if *Vivitrol*™ is given without prior detoxification. Moreover, this drug is very expensive, currently costing ~$1300 for one month. *Vivitrol*™ is being heavily marketed, by pointing out to law enforcement groups, policy-makers, and state legislatures that, unlike buprenorphine and methadone, *Vivitrol*™ has no street value. (83) At the present time, experience with *Vivitrol*™ is limited.

It is imperative that medication-assisted treatment of opioid addiction, whether using methadone, buprenorphine, or naltrexone, is expanded. However, Nicholas Kristof wrote in a *New York Times* Op-Ed column in 2017 that the Secretary of Health and Human Services "seemed to belittle the medication treatments for opioid addiction that have the best record" and the Attorney General "seems to think we can jail our way out of the [opioid abuse and addiction] problem." (70) Nevertheless, there are reasons to be encouraged. The FDA has announced efforts to increase acceptance and availability of medication-assisted treatment for opioid addiction. (84) Both the US House of Representatives and Senate continue to work on legislation to address opioid abuse and addiction.

At a Senate Subcommittee hearing which I attended in December 2017, Dr. Francis Collins, Director of the National Institutes of Health, emphasized the value of medication-assisted treatment for addiction and urged more spending on research into drug addiction, as well as more spending on development of new non-addictive pain medications. (85) At this hearing, Senator Patrick Leahy described how Medicaid dollars, which are a primary source of funding for treatment of addiction and mental illness in the United States, are being successfully used to address opioid addiction in his home state of Vermont. (85) However, current spending by the federal government on treatment of opioid abuse disorder is very limited and substantially below that spent on the recent Zika and Ebola epidemics, as pointed out by Senator Patty Murray of Washington State. (85) Senator Murray advocated for increased funds to treat opioid addiction, as the opioid crisis continues.

In 2018, a House panel and the Senate Health, Education, Labor and Pensions Committee approved a variety of proposals for new opioid legislation. (86) The 2018 fiscal year Omnibus from the House Committee on Appropriations provided nearly four billion dollars to address the opioid crisis. (87) This bill included additional funding for research and for treatment of opioid addiction, although a significant portion was also directed toward enhancing law enforcement. (87) Hopefully, a comprehensive bill, which provides adequate funding for both treatment and research, will be approved and signed into law in the near future.

CONCLUSION

Most people in the medical community agree that prescription opioids are the most effective existing medications to relieve moderate and severe acute pain. The use of opioids for chronic pain relief is more controversial. Additional clinical studies in well-defined patient populations are needed to evaluate the long-term effectiveness of opioids to relieve chronic pain.

In spite of their benefits, opioids are easily abused. Multiple factors have contributed to the current opioid abuse crisis in the United States. However, the media often emphasize the problems of opioids without also describing the pain-relieving benefit that prescription opioids provide to many people. Multiple recent studies have shown that the risk of addiction by patients responsibly taking prescription opioids for pain relief is quite low, and certainly lower than the media would suggest.

But fear of using opioids for pain relief has resulted in increased regulation of prescription opioids, which is negatively impacting patients who truly need opioids to relieve their pain. Many physicians today are reluctant to prescribe these medications. This chapter emphasizes the need for balance between legitimate concerns about opioid abuse and the right of pain patients to have adequate access to prescription opioids. Recent research shows promise in developing new opioid products which enable pain relief but reduce the potential for abuse.

Opioid abuse is a public health problem, not primarily a criminal issue. People who are addicted to opioids are completely preoccupied with obtaining these drugs and will use any method, no matter if illegal or harmful, to obtain them. Opioid addiction is a serious chronic disease, not a moral failure. The brain chemistry of the addicted individual has changed. New approaches to treat opioid addiction with medications show considerable promise. As with other chronic diseases resulting from abnormal biochemistry and physiology, it is likely that long-term treatment with medication is needed for opioid addiction. The current stigma of using medications to treat opioid addiction must be removed. Discussion about the roots of opioid abuse and addiction, which include mental illness, poverty, and lack of job opportunities, is beyond the scope of this book, but such causes of the opioid crisis cannot be remedied through more restrictions on availability of prescription opioids.

CHAPTER 8

―――❧❧❧―――

RECENT RESEARCH TO IDENTIFY NEW PAIN MEDICATIONS

Numerous technological advancements in the latter part of the 20th century enabled scientific discoveries in multiple disciplines, including medicine. Use of the new technologies brought greater understanding about the biochemistry of pain transmission and provided potential opportunities to identify new pain medicines substantially different from the current NSAIDs and opioids.

The pharmaceutical industry has devoted considerable effort to discover and develop new medications for pain relief, but with only limited success to date. Most of the new pain medications that have entered the marketplace are simply improvements upon existing medications, primarily different formulations of older drugs. *Celebrex*™ for relief of inflammatory pain is one of the few new medications consisting of a novel compound (see Chapter 6).

Several so-called new medications to relieve neuropathic pain are drugs that had been previously approved to treat other disorders such as epilepsy.

So, how do researchers discover truly new pain-relieving medicines consisting of novel compounds with a different mechanism of action? One approach is based on plants/medicinal herbs or other "natural products" reported to have pain-relieving properties. Indeed, as described in Chapter 6, two of the pain relievers commonly used today had their origins in plants; specifically, aspirin from willow tree bark/leaves, and opioids from poppies. Recently there has been renewed interest in studying natural products as the basis to discover new pain-relieving medications. Another approach is to study the rare individuals who are insensitive to pain due to genetic disorders. Understanding the cause of these disorders may lead to new avenues for discovering medications to relieve pain. This chapter includes examples of both approaches. However, before describing specific research areas, I need to introduce some general comments about modern drug discovery.

MODERN DRUG DISCOVERY

Medications act by binding to certain molecules, classified as receptors, ion channels, or enzymes, found in various parts of the body. Interactions of the medication with its binding sites can elicit profound biological effects. But some medications interact with more than one type of site and can cause multiple effects. Moreover, when a medication contains multiple active compounds, each compound can attach to its own binding site(s). Historically, most medications were extracts from plants or other natural sources and contained multiple, often poorly defined compounds in varying amounts. Some "natural" medications found in health food stores today are also extracts from a variety of sources and consist of multiple compounds. As a result, these medications may have the desired effect; e.g., pain relief, but also significant side effects (Figure 1A).

Modern FDA standards require that new medications consist of well-defined highly pure compounds. But even when a medication contains only a single active compound, it still may have multiple sites of action and multiple effects, as schematized in Figure 1B. In some cases, this can lead to more effective medicines. But often unpleasant or dangerous side effects occur when a medication acts in multiple ways (Figure 1B). Most drug discovery today focuses on identifying new medications which not only are pure well-defined compounds but also have a single primary mechanism of action (Figure 1C). The rationale is that this type of medication would have fewer side effects.

However, recent research has not forgotten that some natural products, especially certain plants, do have pain-relieving proper-ties. Researchers have sought to understand the biochemical mech-anisms for these pain-relieving effects and to use the information

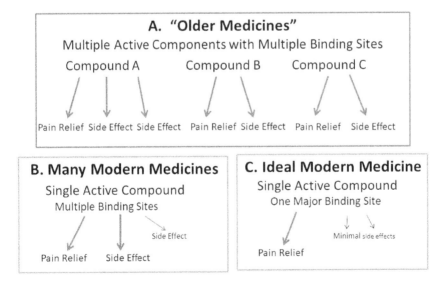

Figure 1. Evolution of Modern Medicines

to guide discovery of new medications. In particular, two types of plants, marijuana and "hot" chili peppers, spawned research efforts to identify new safe and effective pain medications, as discussed in the next two sections of this chapter.

MARIJUANA/CANNABIS

Marijuana, derived from *Cannabis sativa* or *Cannabis indica* plants, has been used for millennia to treat pain and a variety of other disorders. (1) Today, the use of marijuana to relieve pain is a topic of great interest but also controversy. Some states and localities have legalized marijuana for pain relief, but it is still classified as a Schedule I drug by the US federal government and is highly regulated (Chapter 6). As a Schedule I drug, marijuana is in the same category as heroin and LSD, based on the current view by the federal government that marijuana does not have an accepted medical use. Clearly, the Schedule I classification is in conflict with the recent legalization of marijuana for pain relief by many jurisdictions.

Many people find that marijuana does relieve their pain. But anecdotal reports are not sufficient for the standards of modern medications. Clinical trials involving groups of patients are required to draw conclusions about the effectiveness of a particular medication. Importantly, the pain-relieving effects of marijuana and its components, known collectively as cannabinoids, have been studied in a few clinical trials. A review of these combined clinical studies found "moderate quality evidence" that marijuana/cannabis and cannabinoids can relieve chronic pain. (2) Another review reported that some cannabinoids had a small analgesic effect on chronic neuropathic pain. (3) A mixture of cannabinoids, sold under the name *Sativex®*, is available as an oral spray for treatment of multiple sclerosis, and to some extent cancer pain, in Europe and Canada. But it is not currently approved in the US. (4, 5)

In contrast, an extensive review in 2018 concluded that "It

seems unlikely that cannabinoids are highly effective medicines for chronic noncancer pain." (6, 7) However, this review lumped together the overall effects of cannabinoids on patients with many types of chronic pain. Therefore, it does not rule out that cannabinoids may be effective in relieving *some* types of chronic pain. (7)

Clearly, more research is needed on the potential for cannabinoids to relieve chronic pain. In the evolution of modern pain medicines, *Cannabis* extracts can be categorized as an "older medicine" (Figure 1A). Indeed, *Cannabis* plants contain more than 60 pharmacologically active compounds. (4) The contribution of each of these to pain relief is not well understood. Since extracts from *Cannabis* plants can vary in their method of preparation, they may have different composition, leading to differing degrees of effectiveness in pain relief and differing side effects.

Researchers have sought to identify the main pain-relieving components of marijuana and have found that δ–9-tetrahydrocannabinol (THC) is one of the major ingredients. However, THC also has powerful psychoactive effects. As a result, THC and its analogs have not been approved by the FDA for pain relief, although they are approved for relief of severe nausea and vomiting resulting from cancer chemotherapy. (4,8) THC can be categorized as one of several modern medications, consisting of a single compound with multiple sites of action, as depicted in Figure 1B.

Recent cannabinoid research has focused on learning more about the biochemical mechanisms behind the pain-relieving effects of cannabinoids and then utilizing this knowledge to identify new compounds that could relieve pain but not have the euphoria associated with marijuana and most cannabinoids.

Several years ago, it was discovered that THC binds and activates at least two types of receptors, known as cannabinoid receptors 1 and 2 (CB1 and CB2). CB1 receptors were found in many parts of the body, including the brain, whereas CB2 receptors were thought to have a more restricted location, primarily in immune cells outside the brain. (9) Based on these observations, it was hypothesized that a drug which selectively activated CB2 receptors would provide pain relief but not have the pronounced psychoactive effects of THC and marijuana that occurred by activating CB1 receptors in the brain. (9) Such a hypothetical modern medicine is depicted in Figure 1C.

Compounds known as CB2 agonists, which selectively activate CB2 receptors, have been identified and shown to reduce pain in a variety of preclinical animal models. (10, 11) Unfortunately, clinical studies to date with the selective CB2 agonists have been disappointing. (10) One CB2 agonist is reportedly in clinical trials for pain associated with inflammatory bowel disease and irritable bowel syndrome (12), although no results have been reported at the time of writing this chapter.

There are several possible reasons why the selective CB2 agonists have not yet lived up to their promise of relieving human pain. Even though the CB2 agonists block pain in animal models, species differences may account for the poor pain relief in human clinical trials. It is also possible that the original hypothesis was flawed, since there have been difficulties in definitively determining the contributions of each cannabinoid receptor type to pain relief. (9, 10) Interestingly, a non-selective CB1/CB2 agonist, which cannot enter the brain, reportedly relieved pain in animal models by activating the *CB1* receptors in the periphery, not the CB2 receptors. (13) Perhaps the answer to an effective and safe drug is not CB2 selectivity after all!

Another reason may be the complex cellular response which occurs after activation of CB2 receptors. (9, 10) There is still much to learn about cannabinoids and their role in pain relief. Perhaps CB2 agonists can be optimized to produce some but not all of the cellular responses. New compounds have been reported to activate

CB2 receptors differently from previous CB2 agonists. One of these compounds blocks neuropathic pain in rodents (14), but it is not currently known whether it can be successfully developed into a new medication.

CAPSAICIN RECEPTOR

Another type of pain research that also originated with known properties of plants is based on a compound known as capsaicin, which is found in chili peppers. Capsaicin produces the relatively short-lived "hot" burning feeling in the mouth that accompanies eating chilis.

A synthetic form of capsaicin, known as CNTX-4975, is being developed by Centrexion Therapeutics as a new medication for pain relief. You may ask: why is a compound that *generates* a painful feeling being developed as a medication to *relieve* pain? The answer is that after causing the initial burning sensation, capsaicin and related compounds inactivate the nerve fibers that transmit the pain signal. Based on the hypothesis that inactivation of these nerve fibers would relieve chronic pain, a study was performed in which CNTX-4975 was injected directly into the knees of patients with osteoarthritis. Prior to the injection, patients received other medications or ice packs to blunt the initial pain produced by CNTX-4975 itself. The study demonstrated that injection of CNTX-4975 did substantially reduce ongoing knee pain. (15, 16) Moreover, the pain relief was reported to continue for at least six months after a single injection. (16) Due to the urgent need for better pain medications, the FDA gave CNTX-4975 "fast-track status" in 2018 to expedite its development. Advanced clinical trials of CNTX-4975 for osteoarthritis knee pain are ongoing. (16)

Another approach to developing new medications for pain relief involves blocking, instead of first activating, the capsaicin receptor known as TRPV1. A compound which blocks a receptor, rather than activating it, is known as an antagonist. A TRPV1 antagonist would avoid the initial pain caused by capsaicin or CNTX-4975 and could be administered as an oral pill. But you may ask, why would blocking TRPV1 be expected to relieve human clinical pain? Obviously, the goal of such a drug isn't to block the burning sensation caused by eating chili peppers! The answer is that many molecules normally present in our bodies activate TRPV1, resulting in pain (see Chapter 1, Figure 5). (17, 18) TRPV1 has been called an integrator of many pain-generating signals. The hypothesis is that a TRPV1 antagonist would alleviate the pain that occurs in many clinical conditions.

Several pharmaceutical companies, including the company where I worked, competed to identify the most effective, safest TRPV1 antagonist and then move the best compound forward for clinical development. Many TRPV1 antagonists were identified. (19, 20) These antagonists did block activation of TRPV1 by multiple pain-inducing stimuli and reduced pain in animal models of several types of pain. (17, 21, 22)

One of these TRPV1 antagonists was a compound called ABT-102. When I was Director of Neuroscience and Pain Research at Abbott Laboratories (now AbbVie), my responsibilities included overseeing preclinical studies of ABT-102 and other TRPV1 antagonists, as well as research on additional receptors and ion channels involved in pain transmission. We found that ABT-102 potently blocked activation of TRPV1 and had analgesic effects in animal models of inflammatory pain, bone cancer pain, and osteoarthritis pain. (22) Interestingly, repeated dosing of ABT-102 increased the pain-relieving effect. (22) No significant preclinical safety, toxicology, or pharmacology issues prevented the start of human studies.

As is customary in clinical trials of new medications, the first human studies of ABT-102 evaluated the concentrations achieved in plasma and determined how long the compound stayed in circulation after oral dosing. The results supported moving forward to evaluate the effects of ABT-102 in clinical studies on human pain.

Experimental pain models have been developed to study new pain medications in human volunteers (see Chapter 10). In these studies, pain sensitivity is increased through a variety of methods to mimic the clinical conditions of inflammatory or neuropathic pain. (23)

We found that ABT-102 *did* reduce pain generated by application of heat to mildly inflamed skin in an experimental human pain model. (24) A competitor's TRPV1 antagonist (called SB-705498) also decreased pain caused by applying heat to a site of inflammation. (25) These results were encouraging, since they demonstrated that TRPV1 antagonists could indeed block inflammatory pain in humans, consistent with the preclinical animal studies.

However, as human clinical studies continued, warning signs began to emerge. The first concern was the observation that TRPV1 antagonists elevated the body temperature of the volunteers. (26) The extent and duration of the elevated temperature varied with different TRPV1 antagonists. (26) With ABT-102, the average increase in body temperature was approximately 1°C after a single dose. (27) To our relief, the elevated temperature did not continue. After repeated dosing of ABT-102 for four days, body temperature returned to normal. (27)

But a more serious safety concern also arose in these early human studies. We found that ABT-102 decreased pain sensitivity not only on sites of inflammation but also on normal skin. (24) Competitors' TRPV1 antagonists had similar effects. (25, 26) In some respects, these results from the human studies were surprising. Various earlier preclinical studies had yielded conflicting conclusions about whether TRPV1 antagonists would blunt normal sensation of pain in the absence of inflammation. (28-30) Our preclinical studies with ABT-102 and other TRPV1 antagonists had shown only minor, if any, effects on normal pain sensation in rodents in the absence of inflammation. (18, 21, 22)

More extensive clinical studies were performed to better evaluate this safety concern. These follow-up studies confirmed that ABT-102 did decrease heat sensitivity on both normal and inflamed skin. Moreover, when the volunteers were given a hot liquid to drink, they underestimated how hot the liquid actually was. (27) Unfortunately, unlike the normalization of elevated body temperature, the decreased sensitivity to heat did not diminish after repeated dosing of ABT-102. As a result, there was considerable concern that the decreased heat sensitivity would subject individuals to the danger of getting burned from scalding water, e.g., in the shower, from a hot pan on the stove, or from drinking a very hot cup of coffee.

Due to the temporary impaired temperature regulation and especially the ongoing decreased ability to feel pain when exposed to dangerously high temperatures, further clinical studies of these first TRPV1 antagonists, including ABT-102, were halted.

Clearly there was a significant safety concern if ABT-102 and other early TRPV1 antagonists were approved for administration to the general population. However, perhaps these early TRPV1 antagonists could have been developed to provide pain relief for hospitalized patients, nursing home residents, or other people in controlled environments.

But then, research on TRPV1 antagonists as potential pain-relieving medications moved in a new direction. As shown in Chapter 1 Figure 5, TRPV1 can be directly or indirectly activated by many pain-producing stimuli. We had originally hypothesized that it would be an advantage for a TRPV1 antagonist to block multiple pain-producing stimuli, reasoning that such a compound would have the potential to relieve many types of pain. However, with the discovery of clinical side effects that limited further development of these initial TRPV1 antagonists, we and others hypothesized that perhaps a compound which blocked TRPV1 activation by only some stimuli might provide pain relief without the side effects.

So we, as well as scientists at other pharmaceutical companies, began to look for new TRPV1 antagonists which blocked TRPV1 activation by some, but not all, stimuli. (31-33) One activator of TRPV1 is acid, which is generated at sites of inflammation and plays an important role in inflammatory pain and in bone cancer pain. New TRPV1 antagonists were discovered, which completely blocked activation by several stimuli, but not by acid, and blocked pain in some, but not all, rodent models. Moreover, these new TRPV1 antagonists did not elevate body temperature in rodents and in some cases even lowered body temperature. (31-34)

I am no longer actively involved in pain research. But to my delight, a TRPV1 antagonist known as NEO6860, which blocks TRPV1 activation by capsaicin but not to a major extent by either acid or heat, did enter clinical studies. (35) NEO6860 was championed and developed by the private NEOMED Institute located in Quebec, Canada (36) Unlike the previous TRPV1 antagonists than entered clinical development, NEO6860 reportedly had no effect on either body temperature or the ability to sense noxious heat. (35, 37) These results, coupled with the preliminary report that NEO6860 relieved pain in patients with osteoarthritis of the knee, were exciting and encouraging. (37) No further clinical updates on NEO6860 were available at the time of writing. Perhaps NEO6860 or other compounds, which block TRPV1 activation by only selected stimuli, will effectively alleviate chronic pain without the safety issues associated with the earlier compounds.

SODIUM CHANNELS

Another area of research to discover new medications for pain relief is based on the importance of electricity in pain transmission. As discussed in Chapter 1, neurons are the primary cells in the body which generate the sensation of pain. Neurons are sometimes known as excitable cells. After activation by a variety of stimuli, an electrical current passes through the neuron. The current is generated by the opening of specific channels on the surface of the neuron. These channels enable positively charged ions such as sodium and calcium to enter the cell, thereby generating and transmitting electrical signals. (see Chapter 1, Figure 5)

Neuroscientists have extensively studied sodium channels, which play a primary role in neuronal excitability. Nine distinct sodium channels have been identified and several are important in pain sensation. (38, 39) The well-known local anesthetics novocaine and lidocaine, commonly used by dentists and surgeons, eliminate pain by blocking sodium channels. Patches containing lidocaine are also widely used to reduce other types of localized pain (Chapter 6).

However, the clinical use of lidocaine is limited, since it cannot be administered via a pill. This is in part due to its physical properties, but also because it affects multiple types of sodium channels. These include not only the sodium channels involved in pain, but also the sodium channels that are essential for muscle contraction and cardiac function. As a result, there would be major safety issues if lidocaine were present at high concentrations throughout the body.

As discussed earlier in this chapter, modern drug discovery is based on identifying new medicines which have only one or a few well-defined sites/mechanisms of action. As a result, researchers have looked for compounds which selectively block one or only a few types of sodium channels that are primarily found on neurons involved in pain transmission.

One type of sodium channel known as Nav1.7 has attracted considerable attention in pain research. (38, 39) Nav1.7 is expressed on peripheral nerves involved in pain transmission but *not* in the heart or muscles. Moreover, Nav1.7 is *required* for pain transmission. This is an important point, since pain is highly complex with many types of molecules (including neurotransmitters, receptors, ion channels, enzymes) in pain transmission pathways, resulting in some redundancy. Modulating the activity of one of these molecules does not always relieve pain.

However, the situation is different with Nav1.7. There are some individuals who do not feel pain at all, due to rare mutations in the Nav1.7 channel which make it nonfunctional. (40, 41) In contrast, there are other Nav1.7 mutations which have the opposite effect; people with such mutations have severe, ongoing painful conditions. (40, 41) Both types of inherited human conditions clearly demonstrate the importance of Nav1.7 in pain transmission.

As a result, several biotech and pharmaceutical companies initiated research programs to identify compounds which selectively block Nav1.7. One of these compounds, known as XEN-402 or TV-45070, was evaluated as a new topical pain medication. Although early clinical trials seemed promising, the compound did not significantly reduce pain in later studies in patients with osteoarthritis or post-herpetic neuralgia. (42, 43)

Another Nav1.7 inhibitor CNV1014802 (44) entered clinical trials for several types of neuropathic pain. Unfortunately, development of this compound, also known as BIIB074 and vixotrigine, (45) was discontinued for sciatic nerve pain late in 2018. It is not currently known if development is continuing for other types of pain.

NERVE GROWTH FACTOR

During early human development, a molecule known as Nerve Growth Factor (NGF) plays a major role in growth and survival of neurons. In adults, NGF is primarily involved in pain transmission. (46) Increased amounts of NGF are present in a variety of painful conditions. Based on this and other evidence that NGF is an important player in pain transmission, there have been multiple efforts to generate new pain medications which block the action of NGF. (47) One approach has been to develop antibodies that bind to NGF (anti-NGF mAbs), preventing NGF from acting. (46, 47)

Tanezumab is one of the anti-NGF mAbs that entered human clinical studies. Very promising early results were obtained. Tanezumab substantially reduced knee pain in patients with moderate-to-severe osteoarthritis. (48, 49) Side effects were initially reported to be low. (49) But unfortunately, many patients who had received tanezumab subsequently developed *worsening* osteoarthritis, even to the point of needing total joint replacements. In 2010 the FDA placed a hold on further clinical trials of tanezumab and other anti-NGF mAbs. (47)

The hold was finally lifted in 2015. (50) Clinical trials of tanezumab and another anti-NGF mAb, called fasinumab, resumed. (51) Reviews published in 2017 stated that the anti-NGF mAbs substantially relieved pain in many patients with osteoarthritis, although clearly there were safety issues. (51, 52) In late 2019, Pfizer reported results from an advanced clinical study. This study found that tanezumab did significantly improve pain and function in many OA patients. (53) However, some patients who received anti-NGF mAbs exhibited worsening of their OA. (51-54) Recently, Regeneron stated that they have identified a safe dose of fasinumab, which appears to be continuing in advanced studies. (54, 55) It is not currently known whether an anti-NGF mAb can eventually be developed into an FDA-approved medication to relieve pain.

ONGOING OPIOID RESEARCH

As is well known, opioid abuse and addiction are major public health problems today. But opioids have additional liabilities, even when they are appropriately used to relieve pain. Although opioids may be the most effective medications to relieve severe pain, many people choose not to take opioids due to severe constipation. Another major liability is the risk of respiratory depression. This risk increases with high doses and is the major limitation to the amount administered in the hospital or prescribed by a doctor. It is the inability to breathe that causes death from an opioid overdose.

So, even though the current prescription opioids are far from perfect medications, they still are the most effective medications to relieve severe pain. As a result, some researchers today are attempting to exploit the complexity of opioid receptor activation to develop a better medication. (56-58) Perhaps a compound which activates some, but not all, of the cellular responses that occur after binding to the major opioid receptor would retain the pain-relieving properties of current prescription opioids but lack at least some of the liabilities. (56-58)

Based on this hypothesis, researchers identified a compound known as TRV130 which binds to the major opioid receptor but activates only some of the cellular responses. (58) After IV injection in initial clinical studies, TRV130 produced rapid pain relief in patients experiencing moderate-to-severe acute pain following surgical removal of bunions. (59) Moreover, TRV130 may have generated even better pain relief than morphine, with greater tolerability. (59) Based on the encouraging results in multiple clinical studies, the FDA granted "Breakthrough Therapy Status" to TRV130, now known as Oliceridine, enabling faster FDA review. (60) In October 2018, Trevena (the company developing Oliceridine) delivered their data package to the FDA for review. The data demonstrated pain relief similar to morphine in two types of surgical studies. Trevena also reported that Oliceridine had a "favorable respiratory safety profile compared with conventional IV opioids." (61) However, the FDA declined to approve Oliceridine in November 2018, requesting additional data. In 2019, Trevena reported promising results from advanced studies in patients with moderate-to-severe acute pain. (62) Current status of Oliceridine is unknown. However, research is ongoing to discover better opioid medications, by attempting to exploit the complexities of opioid receptors and mechanisms of action.(63, 64)

OTHER ONGOING RESEARCH

Multiple types of research are ongoing to identify new medications for pain. It is beyond the scope of this book to discuss all of them, but one recent publication in the journal *Science* particularly caught my attention. The article described studies which are focused not on the physical sensation of pain, but rather the emotional aspect of pain. These studies identified circuits in the brain which are responsible for the unpleasantness of pain. Perhaps this information could eventually lead to new ways to relieve pain by decreasing the unpleasantness of pain without blocking normal sensations of noxious stimuli. These early studies performed in mice are obviously a long way from gaining FDA approval for a new pain medication. Nevertheless, the discovery is intriguing and will likely generate further research. (65, 66)

WHY SO LITTLE PROGRESS?

The failure rate of potential new pain medications in human clinical trials is very high. Why has there been so little progress, in spite of the increased scientific understanding of pain? No doubt there are many reasons, including the overall complexity of pain transmission and perception. The section in this chapter on cannabinoids discusses some possible reasons for the disappointing clinical results. Several additional reasons have also been proposed. (9, 10) These include irrelevance of the animal pain models; inadequate selectivity for a particular receptor, ion channel or enzyme being targeted; inability of the new compound to reach adequate concentrations in the tissues involved in pain; side effects/safety issues not detected in preclinical studies; failure to evaluate the new medication in the appropriate type of human clinical pain.

Rodent pain models are used to evaluate potential new pain medications prior to human clinical studies. But animal models of pain are artificial and can't truly mimic chronic human pain, such as osteoarthritis and neuropathic pain. (67) Moreover, due to species differences, compounds which decrease pain in rodents may not relieve pain in humans. (9, 10) Even when a receptor or ion channel is *almost* identical in rodents and humans, there are always some differences. Seemingly minor species differences may have profound effects.

It is useful to mention that mice have been genetically engineered in which the human equivalent of a particular receptor or enzyme has replaced its mouse counterpart. Studying potential new medications in these mice can enhance confidence that the medication will act on the human receptor or enzyme. However, species differences can continue to play a role, since the rest of the animal is still a mouse, not a human. (10)

The first human clinical trials of potential new pain medications are usually conducted in acute painful conditions, such as dental pain or after surgical removal of bunions. These clinical studies are relatively inexpensive and can rapidly determine whether the new compounds are effective in relieving acute inflammatory pain. In contrast, clinical trials for chronic pain are very expensive. If a new compound is not very effective in the initial clinical studies in acute pain, the compound may never progress to the more expensive studies in patients with chronic neuropathic or osteoarthritic pain. As a result, there could be a missed opportunity to discover whether this compound could actually become a breakthrough new medication to relieve chronic pain.

CONCLUSION

I apologize that some of this chapter reads as a scientific review article. But I hope that the descriptions of various research efforts provide insight into the challenges in discovering truly new and better pain-relieving medications. Each research endeavor consists of its own opportunities but also difficulties and hurdles. Unfortunately, most research areas, which begin with great optimism based on scientific advances and preclinical studies, do not yield breakthrough new drugs. A statement on the office door of Dr. Joost Oppenheim, who was my mentor at the National Cancer Institute, reads "another beautiful hypothesis ruined by an ugly fact." Although these ugly facts are always disappointing, it is better if they come early in a research project. Unfortunately, the ugly facts are often only revealed later in clinical development.

Drug discovery and development are difficult endeavors in all therapeutic areas. But discovering and developing new pain medications is especially difficult. This is particularly true for chronic pain, which requires long and expensive clinical trials. Also, there are understandably high safety requirements for medications that will be used by patients long-term to relieve chronic pain.

This chapter describes recent efforts, along with disappointments, in the quest for better medications to relieve pain. Hopefully the ongoing work, including the compounds currently in development, will lead to new and better pain medications. Scientific understanding of pain continues to grow and presents new opportunities. The research areas described are only a few of the various efforts in academia and the pharmaceutical industry to discover and develop better pain medications.

I end this chapter with a quote from the late Senator Edward Kennedy in a concession speech ending his campaign in 1980 for nomination as the Democratic presidential candidate. "For all those whose cares have been our concern, the work goes on, the cause endures, the hope still lives, and the dream shall never die." (68) To me, this statement is also relevant to the ongoing work to identify new medications which can help relieve the problem of human pain and suffering. The final chapter in this book describes hope for a future in which better pain relief will indeed exist and be widely available.

CHAPTER 9

⸺⁓⸺

ALTERNATIVE METHODS TO MANAGE PAIN

Instead of taking medications, many people today are using other methods to manage their pain. Such alternative approaches have gained popularity due to the problems of opioid abuse and the limited pain relief provided by many other medicines. Alternative methods include chiropractic manipulation, exercise, massage, acupuncture, meditation, behavioral modification, and various types of electrical stimulation. There is increasing evidence that these approaches do relieve pain for some individuals. A 2018 report concluded that several of the alternative approaches can have a "small net health benefit" when added to "usual care." (1) This chapter briefly describes some of the alternative methods to relieve pain, focusing on current scientific understanding of how they may provide pain relief for some people.

SPINAL MANIPULATION AND EXERCISE

Many individuals suffering from back or neck pain undergo spinal manipulation primarily by a chiropractor to relieve their pain. (2, 3) A 2017 review of 26 randomized clinical trials found that spinal manipulative therapy; i.e., chiropractic treatment, had statistically significant, but modest benefits in reducing pain and improving function in patients with acute low back pain. (3) But more than half of the patients who received spinal manipulative therapy experienced minor, short-lived side effects such as increased pain, muscle stiffness, and headache. (3)

An editorial accompanying the review stated that in spite of its current popularity, chiropractic treatment remains controversial and is not widely accepted by many traditional health care providers. (4) Many physicians have viewed spinal manipulation as quackery and potentially dangerous. Nevertheless, adding chiropractic treatment to usual medical care has been shown to produce statistically significant "moderate short-term improvements in low back pain intensity and disability in active-duty military personnel." (5) Additional studies in other patient populations with chronic back pain would be insightful.

Exercise is often recommended to relieve chronic low back pain. In particular, a regimen known as lumbar extensor strengthening, which utilizes progressive increases in resistance, can be effective. (6) One study has concluded that a structured exercise program appears to be as effective as chiropractic treatment for patients with chronic low back pain. (7) Physical therapy can also relieve pain for some, but certainly not all, people. (8)

ACUPUNCTURE

Acupuncture has been used for millennia in China and other Asian countries to treat a variety of ailments, including pain. (9) In the early 1970s, the Western world began to take notice of the ability of acupuncture to relieve pain. While accompanying the US Secretary of State Henry Kissinger on an historic trip to China in 1971, the *New York Times* reporter James Reston had an emergency appendectomy. After his surgery, Reston received acupuncture treatment for relief of gastrointestinal pain. He wrote about his experience and stated that acupuncture relieved his discomfort. (10) Subsequently, acupuncture began to gain some acceptance in the US, especially for low back pain and other painful musculoskeletal conditions. According to one survey, 8 million adults in the US have used acupuncture, primarily for chronic pain. (9) However, many Western physicians remain skeptical.

We now have some understanding of how properly conducted acupuncture may relieve pain. Acupuncture needles are thought to activate specific peripheral nerves, resulting in short-term release of natural pain-relieving molecules both in the periphery and in the spinal cord or brain. Acupuncture may also cause long-term changes in the body. For example, acupuncture therapy of individuals with hand pain has been reported to change the thickness of specific regions of the brain associated with pain relief. (11, 12)

ELECTRICAL STIMULATION

Peripheral nerve stimulation is also the basis for some other therapies to relieve pain. In one method, known as transcutaneous electrical stimulation (TENS), electrodes are used to stimulate peripheral nerves. TENS has been utilized to some extent since the early 1970s, but its application was limited until a small nerve stimulator was approved by the FDA in 2014. This device, known as *Quell*™, is discrete and easy to use. It is small enough to be worn on the upper calf. (13, 14) One study has found that *Quell*™ decreased pain in 81% of the patients with chronic low back and lower extremity pain. (14)

Another electrical stimulation method to reduce chronic pain is known as scrambler therapy. This method utilizes small device-containing pads, which are placed around the painful area and then activated to produce non-painful stimulation of peripheral nerves. A device employing this technology, known as *Calmare®*, has been approved for use in the US and Europe. (15) It is thought that these devices replace the pain transmission signals with non-painful signals; in effect, scrambling the pain signals. (15) Perhaps a similar scrambling of signals from nerves also contributes to pain relief obtained with acupuncture.

Scrambler therapy has been reported to relieve many types of pain; in particular, chemotherapy-induced neuropathic pain in cancer patients. In one study, cancer patients at the Mayo Clinic indicated that their chemotherapy-induced pain was significantly reduced after ten consecutive days of scrambler therapy. A 53% reduction in average pain scores and a 44% decrease in tingling sensations were reported. Moreover, the effect lasted at least ten weeks with no substantial adverse effects. (15, 16) The senior author of this publication stated that it takes a long time for practitioners to learn how to perform the technique effectively, but he expected that eventually it will become more widely used for many types of chronic pain. (15)

In addition to electrical stimulation of painful peripheral areas of the body, stimulation of the brain also shows promise in relieving some types of pain. There are two basic types of brain stimulation techniques: repetitive transcranial magnetic stimulation (rTMS) and transcranial direct-current stimulation (tCDS). Both of these non-invasive techniques are still in the experimental stage for pain management.

As the name implies, rTMS uses a magnetic coil which is placed on the scalp. Stimulation of the coil creates a short-lived magnetic field that passes through the skull to the brain. As a result, an electrical field is induced in the brain, activating neurons and altering brain signaling. rTMS has been reported to significantly relieve pain for some types of neuropathic pain, especially after multiple treatments. (17, 18) The other brain stimulation method (tCDS) directly applies weak electrical currents to the scalp. These electrical currents supposedly activate or inhibit specific neurons, resulting in a cascade of events to reduce pain. Both technologies provide only temporary relief and there are safety concerns, especially for rTMS. (19)

Another method to manage chronic back and leg pain utilizes spinal cord stimulation. (20, 21) Unlike the techniques described above, this method is invasive and requires surgery. A small battery-operated electrical generator is implanted under the skin in the patient's buttocks or abdomen. Wires from the generator are connected to electrodes that have been surgically placed in the spine. The patient then uses a remote control to activate the generator, which sends an electrical stimulus to the spine. As a result, the pain sensation is reduced. The stimulus also produces a temporary tingling feeling, which some people find very uncomfortable, although less noxious than the underlying pain. Spinal cord stimulation has been reported to relieve multiple types of neuropathic pain and to be more effective than current medications for patients with intractable spine or limb pain. (22) Many patients, including a close personal friend, say that this technology has substantially relieved their pain and improved their mobility. In one study, spinal cord stimulation continued to be effective over a five-year follow-up period for patients with painful diabetic neuropathy. (23) But the therapy does not appear effective in relieving musculoskeletal pain, such as arthritis pain. (22)

NERVE ABLATION

Early in 2019, the FDA approved another alternative approach to relieve chronic pain. Instead of stimulating nerves in the methods just described, this technology selectively destroys nervous tissue. This minimally invasive system, called *Accurian*™, uses radio frequency to ablate a small area of nervous tissue so that it can no longer transmit pain signals. (24) *Accurian*™ is highly flexible and can produce a range of sizes and shapes of the lesions, enabling a pain specialist to target the relevant nervous tissue. (24) *Accurian*™ provides another tool for pain specialists to relieve chronic pain. It will be interesting to see whether it will be utilized only in highly specialized pain clinics or will gain more widespread use for patients who have not had their chronic pain controlled by medications or other alternative methods.

PAIN CLINICS AND BEHAVIORAL MODIFICATION

The establishment of specialized pain clinics is a relatively new development in pain management. Some clinics utilize both medications and alternative methods to manage chronic pain. Others, such as the Pain Rehabilitation Center at the Mayo Clinic in Minnesota, emphasize use of the alternative non-pharmacological methods. (25) The director of this pain clinic is a clinical psychologist with a specialty in behavioral pain management. The clinic focuses on improving the quality of life of chronic pain patients, especially functional capability, without relying on medications such as opioids to relieve pain. Patients in the program must first taper off any pain medications they are taking. In an interview with National Public Radio, the clinical director said that the Mayo Clinic's pain center takes a biopsychosocial approach, which emphasizes the impact of mood, anxiety, and other factors on an individual's pain perception. (25)

The Mayo Clinic and many other pain clinics use something called behavioral modification to manage chronic pain. This method is based on the concept that much of the suffering from pain is due to learned behaviors, and therefore changing one's behavior can diminish the suffering. A pioneer in the field of behavioral modification to manage chronic pain is the clinical psychologist Wilbert Fordyce, who published an influential book on the topic in 1976. (26, 27) He also founded the University of Washington Multidisciplinary Pain Clinic, which was one of the first US clinics to incorporate cognitive-behavioral therapy (CBT) into pain management. CBT theories and practice have expanded following the pioneering work of Fordyce. Various forms of CBT, including biofeedback, are often part of the multidisciplinary approach used today in pain clinics. (28)

We now have some understanding of how CBT may relieve pain. Emotional stress and anxiety caused by pain can lead to increased levels of stress molecules such as adrenaline and cortisol. These molecules enhance nerve conductivity and as a result magnify pain sensations. CBT may reduce anxiety and consequently reduce the overproduction of pain-enhancing molecules. (28) Although CBT can help manage chronic pain, it is not a cure-all. It is often most effective when combined with other pain-relieving methods.

From my perspective, some clinicians have over-emphasized the psychological and behavioral aspects of pain and suffering. For example, Dr. Steven F Brena published a book entitled *Pain and Religion: A Psychophysiologic Study*. (29) The author's thesis is that pain is a point of convergence between medical science and religion. He emphasizes the impact of psychology and personal behavior on chronic pain. (29) Although pain sensation certainly has psychological components, considering *only* the psychological and behavioral aspects of pain has a dark side, since it seems dangerously close to earlier centuries when individuals were blamed for their pain and suffering (Chapters 2 and 3). Indeed, Brena wrote in his book that mental illness and pain either are punishments and/or are meant to be "handled." (30) He stated that pain is a habit or a behavior which children quickly learn in order to escape from threatening or unpleasant situations. He went on to write that what we call "chronic pain and suffering" are actually distorted behaviors, resulting from failure to monitor emotions when exposed to noxious sensations. (30) Certainly, such words appear to blame the individual for his pain and suffering; i.e., if a patient feels and acknowledges pain, it is his own fault. The implication is that if only he would change his behavior, the problem would go away. Too much suffering has occurred through the ages from such a perspective!

Nevertheless, many pain clinics do emphasize the psychological aspects of pain, including the use of behavioral modification. In 2018, two psychiatrists wrote that CBT can effectively treat chronic pain, either alone or with only mild pain-relieving medications. (31) They emphasized that CBT improves the quality of life and mobility of pain patients. (31) In an interview with *Medscape*, one of the authors stated that physicians should discuss with their patients that day-to-day functioning is "more important than the numbers on the pain scale." (32) Whoa! In other words, how you feel doesn't matter, as long as you can function! Such a viewpoint belittles the significance of ongoing pain experienced by chronic pain sufferers. In addition to CBT, the psychiatrist also discussed another psychological therapy known as acceptance and commitment therapy (ACT). The goal of ACT is to help the patient *accept* suffering. (32) Yes, in earlier times, the only option *was* to accept pain and suffering, but that is not the case today. Indeed, the overall feeling of pain is highly complex and the result of both physical and emotional components (Chapter 1). But the danger comes when only the psychological/emotional aspects of pain are considered and the physical components are belittled. The goal of modern medicine must be to relieve pain for each individual by using the available tools as appropriate and needed.

THE PLACEBO EFFECT AND MINDFULNESS MEDITATION

The complexity of pain sensation is apparent in a well-known complication of clinical trials for new pain medications: the placebo effect. Clinical trials often compare the pain relief reported by patients receiving the new drug with that reported by those who did not receive the drug, but instead received a dummy pill known as a placebo. The trials are conducted in a blinded manner, so that neither the patients nor the clinicians know who received the drug and who received the placebo. Interestingly, patients who received only the placebo often report significant pain relief! The placebo effect can occur not only with dummy pills but also with non-medicinal creams and with sham acupuncture.

The placebo effect on pain relief can be quite pronounced in some individuals. (33) How is this possible? One way is via opioids made by our own bodies. These opioids are different from the pain-relieving prescription medications such as morphine, oxycodone, and hydrocodone. In the 1970s, it was discovered that our bodies make other types of opioids, known as endorphins and enkephalins. (34) The molecules are small peptides, which are very different in structure from the opioid medications. Nevertheless, the endorphins and enkephalins block pain transmission in ways similar to opioid medications. (34) The current view is that placebos reduce pain by enhancing levels of the opioids made in the individual's body. (33, 35, 36) As a result, by simply *expecting* pain relief, placebos can actually provide relief at least in part through our own opioids. These molecules may also contribute to the pain relief provided by some nerve stimulation methods (13), described earlier in this chapter.

Imaging studies described in Chapter 10 have shown that placebo-induced pain relief modifies activity in several regions of the brain. (37-39) However, a recent review has concluded that the

major brain regions involved in the placebo effect are *not* those involved in transmitting the pain sensation from the periphery *up to*
the brain. (40) Instead, placebos may act primarily by sending a signal *from* the brain back to the spinal cord, decreasing the excitability of neurons and dampening pain sensation. (38-40) Interestingly,
some brain regions activated by placebos are the same as those
activated by opioid medications. (38)

It has even been suggested that perhaps placebos themselves
could be used as pseudo-medications to relieve pain. There are
clearly ethical issues with placebo use in clinical practice, particularly when used deceptively. (41) Nevertheless, some patients with
chronic musculoskeletal pain may knowingly accept placebos as
one approach to relieve their pain. (42)

Mindfulness meditation, also called mindfulness-based stress
reduction (MBSTR), is used by some individuals to relieve pain. This
approach, which has its origins in Buddhist meditation and yoga,
utilizes focus and concentration to only pay attention to thoughts
and sensations at the moment. In a recent experimental pain study
with healthy volunteers, MBSTR was more effective than a placebo in reducing pain. (43) Interestingly, brain imaging studies have
shown that mindfulness meditation and placebos activated different parts of the brain, suggesting that they relieve pain by different
mechanisms. (43)

CONCLUSION

Currently, there is widespread interest in pain-relieving methods
that do not utilize medications. This chapter describes both biophysical and psychological alternative methods to relieve pain. Biophysical
methods include exercise, spinal manipulation, acupuncture, electrical stimulation, and nerve ablation. Emotions contribute to overall
pain sensation, supporting the role for psychological therapies, such
as behavioral modification and meditation techniques.

The various alternative methods described in this chapter help some people manage their chronic pain. Many self-help books describe relief of chronic pain through lifestyle changes or other alternative non-pharmacological methods. But this is not universally true. Due to the complexity of pain, responses of individuals can vary considerably. There is danger in concluding that non-pharmacological methods *alone* can effectively manage pain for *all* pain sufferers.

Although there is still much more to learn about pain, we now know that there are multiple neurotransmitters, natural opioids, stress hormones, and other molecules which modulate pain sensation. These natural molecules, made in our own bodies, can either increase or decrease the feeling of pain. The relative amounts of stimulating and inhibiting molecules determine the level of pain. Interestingly, not only medications, but also the alternative methodologies, can affect the level of these naturally occurring molecules in our bodies. For example, the ability of CBT and other psychological interventions to relieve pain is likely due, at least in part, to a decrease in the levels of stress hormones. As we continue to learn more, we are finding that some of the biochemical mechanisms utilized by medications to provide pain relief are also the basis for pain relief from non-pharmacological methods. This chapter cites the example of the opioids made by our own bodies which contribute to the pain-relieving effects of placebos. Perhaps these natural opioids also contribute to pain relief provided by some of the other non-pharmacological pain-relieving methods discussed.

I suggest that a better term for the alternative methods described in this chapter would be complementary methods, to be used in combination with medications. Since pain is complex and highly individualized, both medications and these complementary approaches are often needed to effectively alleviate human pain.

CHAPTER 10

THE FUTURE OF PAIN MANAGEMENT

During the late 20th and early 21st centuries, numerous advocacy and professional organizations highlighted the worldwide problem of unrelieved pain. In October 2004, the World Health Organization and the International Association for the Study of Pain declared a "Global Day Against Pain." The theme was "Pain Relief Should Be a Human Right." The US Congress declared 2001 through 2010 as the "Decade of Pain Control and Research."

However, in spite of these efforts to increase awareness of unrelieved pain, the problem of pain is still very much with us. Opioids are still the most effective medications to relieve severe pain although they are frequently abused. The first part of the present chapter summarizes efforts to reduce opioid abuse and to prevent deaths from opioid overdoses. The second part discusses other types of research, in addition to the efforts described in Chapter 8, to improve future pain management.

CAN OPIOID ABUSE BE SIGNIFICANTLY REDUCED THROUGH NEW FORMULATIONS?

Several new formulations aimed at preserving the pain-relieving properties of opioids but reducing their potential for abuse are described in Chapter 7. In particular, EMBEDA® is a promising new technology with reduced abuse potential, particularly for those individuals seeking the "high" obtained by inhaling or injecting opioids. It remains to be seen whether the new technologies will actually reduce opioid abuse. Unfortunately, people addicted to opioids often find ways to subvert abuse-deterrent methodologies. Moreover, many of the current problems with opioid abuse are due to street drugs rather than prescription opioids. New formulations of prescription opioids will not address the problem of illicit drugs. One could even argue that new formulations of prescription drugs, which reduce the potential to get "high," will lead to greater use of street drugs by people seeking the psychoactive effects.

OTHER STEPS TO REDUCE OPIOID ABUSE

Prescription-monitoring systems for controlled substances have been established in almost all states in the United States in an attempt to reduce opioid abuse. The monitoring systems, which use electronic databases to track the prescribing and dispensing of opioids, prevent individuals from obtaining the medications from multiple physicians or pharmacies. Twenty-four states have reported an overall 30% reduction in opioid prescriptions, likely due in part to this type of monitoring. (1) Unfortunately, such systems can lead to reluctance of physicians to prescribe opioids for patients who truly need them for pain relief.

As discussed in Chapter 7, screening pain patients for previous/current drug or alcohol abuse would likely decrease the number of patients who abuse their prescription opioids. Another approach to reduce opioid abuse requires that the patient signs an agreement describing the expectations of both the physician and the patient; e.g., how often the medication will be dispensed and the quantity to be dispensed. Agreements can also include additional ways to reduce abuse, such as determining the types/amounts of opioids in the patient's urine as well as the number of remaining pills during follow-up visits to the physician's office. In addition to reducing the potential for abuse, written agreements may provide some legal protection for the prescribing physicians. These procedures, however, would place an additional burden on health care providers who are being pushed to decrease time spent with each patient.

USE OF NALOXONE TO PREVENT DEATHS FROM OPIOID OVERDOSES

Tragic deaths from opioid overdoses occur daily, but there is a major new initiative to reduce such deaths. This initiative, which is based on the ability of a drug called naloxone to reverse the effects of an opioid overdose, has gained widespread acceptance.

To understand how naloxone works, please see the discussion of agonists and antagonists in Chapter 7. Naloxone is an opioid antagonist, which means that it blocks the effects of opioid agonists such as oxycodone and heroin, among others. Because naloxone is an antagonist, it does not have psychoactive effects and does not have the potential for abuse. If given in a timely manner to an overdose victim, naloxone can save the person's life. Naloxone is now widely available to first responders, such as emergency medical technicians. Sometimes patients themselves, who are taking an opioid agonist such as oxycodone for pain relief, are given a prescription for naloxone. A study at six clinics in San Francisco found that chronic pain patients, who were on long-term opioid therapy and also received prescriptions for naloxone, had 63% fewer visits to emergency departments for overdoses after one year. (2)

In the past, naloxone was available only by prescription from a physician or other health care provider. But recently new initiatives have greatly expanded its availability. (3) Standing orders for naloxone are now available at some pharmacies in most states in the US, eliminating the need for a patient to have an individual prescription to obtain this life-saving medication. (4, 5) In some Canadian provinces, naloxone can be sold as an over-the-counter medication without any type of prescription. In 2019, several states in the US have passed laws and regulations that require a physician to also prescribe naloxone or at least offer a naloxone prescription when prescribing an opioid for pain relief. (6)

At first, naloxone existed only in a form to be injected by a person with at least some medical training. Recent development of a device which is an auto-injector of naloxone is a major advancement. This device, known as *Evzio*™, is easy to use and provides a highly effective way to prevent death from an opioid overdose. (7) It is much like the life-saving epinephrine auto-injector which people with severe allergies carry with them at all times. However, of great concern is the high cost of *Evzio*™. (8) The current retail price in the Washington, DC area for a carton of *Evzio*™ containing two auto-injectors is more than $3,800, although savings programs and discounts are available. The company which markets *Evzio*™ announced in December 2018 that a generic form will be available in 2019 for $178, although at time of writing it is not yet on the market. (9) An easy-to-use nasal spray formulation, known as *Narcan*™, has also been developed. It is reasonably priced at $130 for two sprays. Although this easily used formulation is clearly an advantage, the nasal formulation may not be effective if the victim has depressed breathing, which commonly occurs with an opioid overdose. Both *Narcan*™ and *Evzio*™ can have a significant impact in reducing the current scourge of deaths from opioid overdoses, but only if these naloxone formulations are widely available, especially without prescription and at a reasonable price.

IS THERE A "MAGIC BULLET" WAITING TO BE DISCOVERED?

As discussed throughout the book, opioids are the most effective oral medications to relieve severe pain, but they do have significant issues and side effects. Scientists in academia and pharmaceutical companies have been searching for a new medication that could replace opioids. But what is the likelihood of discovering a new medication which is as effective as opioids in relieving pain, but lacks potential for abuse?

In the late 20th century, scientific knowledge about the physiology and biochemistry of pain transmission increased substantially. At this time, there was considerable optimism that the newly identified receptors, enzymes, and ion channels, which had been found to be important in pain transmission, would lead to the discovery of new medicines to relieve pain. But as discussed in Chapter 8, success has been marginal. To date, no new oral medication has been identified with the effectiveness of opioids for severe pain. Chronic pain sufferers, the pharmaceutical industry, and academic pain researchers are disappointed that more progress has not been made in developing new and better pain-relieving medicines.

Because pain transmission involves many pathways and molecules, one might imagine that there would be multiple ways to block pain transmission. However, like other physiological systems, pain transmission is regulated by checks and balances. Some pain pathways appear to be redundant, which is not surprising considering the importance of pain in protecting against further injury. So, although we now know much more about pain transmission and the many players involved, discovering safe and effective medications that act via the newly discovered mechanisms has been extremely difficult. Most research efforts have led to dead ends. Nevertheless, some biotechnology and pharmaceutical companies are still persevering in the attempt to discover better pain medicines.

Due to the complexities of pain transmission, many scientists today assume that it will not be possible to identify a "magic bullet" medication which would provide effective relief of severe pain without serious side effects. Nevertheless, science does march forward, and what seems impossible today may become possible in the future through new research. Many pain researchers and clinicians currently believe that effective pain management without opioids may require a combination of drugs with differing types of activities. This is analogous to modern treatment of high blood pressure, in which patients often receive more than one type of medication acting by different mechanisms.

BARRIERS TO USE OF ALTERNATIVE METHODS TO RELIEVE PAIN

As discussed in Chapter 9, many people try alternative methods to relieve their pain, and these non-pharmacological approaches do provide relief for some individuals. However, a significant barrier exists to their utilization, since many insurance companies in the United States do not cover these less-established methods. (10) A recent review found significant variation in insurance coverage for alternative methods to relieve low back pain. Physical and occupational therapy were covered by almost all the insurance plans evaluated, whereas coverage for other alternative therapies varied widely. For example, only one-third of the insurance plans covered acupuncture. (11) Expanded insurance coverage for alternative methods could help reduce the problem of unrelieved pain.

EFFORTS TO DEVELOP OBJECTIVE MEASURES OF PAIN

Currently there is no objective way for a clinician to determine the severity of a person's pain (Chapter 5). As a result, pain is often underestimated and therefore undertreated. I believe that development of cost-effective objective ways to measure patients' pain should be a priority for pain research. Methodology which could determine the actual level of an individual's pain would have a substantial effect in improving pain relief and minimizing distrust between patients and their physicians. If available, it is likely that physicians would quickly adopt the new methodologies, since they would help guide the choice of medications and reduce some of the concerns about prescribing opioids.

One possible approach utilizes human experimental pain models, in which heat or external pressure are applied to the skin to evoke mild pain. These models have enhanced our understanding about pain (12) and can be used in development of new pain medications. (13) One model, known as quantitative sensory testing (QST), has provided objective data which confirm fibromyalgia patients' own reports that the pain they feel in response to various stimuli is greater than normal. (14) However, it is generally accepted that current experimental pain models cannot provide an objective assessment of most types of chronic pain which occur spontaneously without an external stimulus.

A major area of medical research today is focused on the most complex organ of the body; i.e., the brain. One aspect of brain research utilizes a variety of imaging technologies, which can be divided into those that evaluate *brain structure* and those that measure *brain activity*. These brain-imaging techniques are described below in the context of their potential for developing an objective method to measure pain.

Magnetic resonance imaging (MRI) is one technique used to study brain structure. MRI studies have revealed striking structural abnormalities in the brains of chronic pain patients. (15-19) For example, patients with fibromyalgia (FM) have less gray matter in some discrete pain-related brain regions, compared with healthy individuals. (20, 21) Patients with chronic low back pain (cLBP) also have structural aberrations in several parts of the brain. These include the gray matter in the thalamus, which is involved in detection of sensations from various parts of the body, and the prefrontal cortex, which plays a role in emotional responses to pain. (22) Altered structures have also been observed in other types of chronic pain and in additional regions of the brain. The structural changes have been called anatomical "brain signatures" for patients with chronic pain. Interestingly, the alterations in brain structures differ in various types of chronic pain, emphasizing the complexity of chronic pain and supporting the conclusion that not all pains are the same. (17)

Recent advances in technology have enabled enhanced analysis of data, using a method known as multivariate pattern analysis (MVPA). This methodology can analyze large data sets and identify patterns associated with specific subgroups. MVPA analysis of MRI data has been reported to distinguish cLBP patients from healthy volunteers with 76% accuracy. (18) The areas of the brain that exhibit structural differences include those known to be generally involved in pain processing, as well as some additional areas that may be unique to cLBP patients. (18)

But which came first: the chronic pain or the structural changes in the brain? That is, did the structural changes cause chronic pain, or did chronic pain cause the structural changes? To date, no studies have been reported which compared brain structure in individual patients before and after the onset of pain, although some studies have shown changes in brain structure as pain progressed from acute to chronic. (23) Interestingly, alleviation of the pain has been reported to reverse structural aberrations (24, 25), supporting the conclusion that chronic pain can cause structural changes in the brain.

Pain affects not only brain structure but also brain activity. The most widely used technique to study brain activity is functional magnetic resonance imaging (fMRI), which indirectly measures brain activity by tracking changes in blood oxygenation levels within the brain. (26) A "neurological signature of physical pain" has been identified, based on enhanced analysis of fMRI data. This neurologic pain signature (NPS) showed changes in activity of brain regions associated with heat-induced pain and could distinguish painful heat from non-painful lower temperatures. Moreover, activity in the NPS decreased following administration of a strong opioid. Such studies provided strong support for the role of the NPS in sensation of at least some types of pain. (27)

The fMRI studies described above evaluated the effect of experimentally induced pain in healthy volunteers. fMRI has also been used in studies on chronic pain patients. For example, in response to pain-generating stimuli, FM patients had abnormally increased activation in brain regions that are involved in the overall sensation of pain. (28-32) FM patients also had activity changes in regions of the brain that appear to be more specific to FM. (33) One fMRI study found the total activity changes could distinguish FM patients from healthy volunteers with 94% specificity. (33) fMRI has also been used to study patients with chronic back pain and postherpetic neuralgia. (34, 35) Interestingly, fMRI showed that some brain regions activated by spontaneous pain were distinct from those activated by experimental heat-evoked pain in patients with chronic back pain and post-herpetic neuralgia. (34, 35) Significantly, treatment of post-herpetic neuralgia patients with the local anesthetic lidocaine modulated the brain activity in the fMRI images, consistent with the decrease in spontaneous pain reported by the patients. (35)

Despite these impressive results from imaging the brains of chronic pain patients, it is generally held by experts in the field that the current technologies are not yet sophisticated enough to be used for diagnosis of most types of chronic pain. No single specific

pain center has been identified in the brain; i.e., multiple brain regions are involved. Various types of chronic pain cause changes in
different parts of the brain. Any pain-associated brain image may
also vary with the origin of the pain.

As discussed throughout the book, the overall sensation of pain
is the result of input from the source of the pain, integration of
pain signals in the brain, as well as other mechanisms which can
either enhance or inhibit pain perception. Emotions, prior experiences, and basic beliefs about pain can also have a profound effect
on an individual's pain perception. Current imaging techniques cannot integrate all the factors which ultimately determine pain intensity. But perhaps in the future, brain imaging will be used to aid in
the diagnosis of chronic pain patients, much as an electrocardiogram (EKG) is now routinely used in detecting cardiac disorders and
X-rays are used to diagnose many conditions. An objective way to
measure pain would certainly have a major impact on the problem
of unrelieved pain.

In addition to the potential for brain imaging to provide a way
for physicians to objectively measure pain and its severity, perhaps
brain imaging could be used in early clinical trials to help determine
the effectiveness of a new pain medication. Clinical trials of new
pain medications currently rely on the individual's self-reported
subjective assessment of the pain level. Use of brain imaging as
an objective read-out could assist in the development of new pain
medications. As discussed briefly in Chapter 9, a major confounder
in clinical trials of new pain medications is the large "placebo effect," in which individuals who receive only an ineffective "dummy
pill" report substantially decreased pain. Due to the placebo effect,
it is often difficult to determine whether a new medication is actually having an analgesic effect through its intended mechanism. A
brain-imaging technique which could separate the placebo effect
from an actual analgesic effect would be a boon to the development

of new pain medications. (36, 37) It is likely that many potentially "good" analgesics have been discarded during development due to the placebo effect. (36-38)

ROLE OF GENETICS IN PAIN AND PAIN RELIEF

Each person has a unique genetic profile based on inheriting genetic information from both parents. An individual's genetic make-up plays a major role in all aspects of the person's life. The recent genomics revolution, which includes sequencing of the entire human genome, may someday significantly improve understanding and treatment of a variety of human maladies, including chronic pain. But the impact of the genomics revolution is still in its infancy.

Genetic testing is being used today in some areas of medicine to assist in diagnosis and choice of treatment for a given patient. Perhaps the best-known genetic testing is in the area of breast cancer, in which the specific types of a gene known as BRCA possessed by an individual can both predict the probability of developing breast cancer and influence the choice of treatment. By comparison, pain is highly complex. Multiple genes contribute to pain, making it difficult to determine the role of genetics in an individual's pain. Nevertheless, the effect of genetics on pain is an ongoing area of research.

More than 20% of patients have been reported to develop chronic pain after surgery. (39) Interestingly, a recent study found that genetic variations of one particular gene known as *BDNF* was associated with increased risk of developing post-surgical chronic pain. (39) Expanding such studies may help identify individuals at high risk for post-surgical chronic pain and lead to more intensive pain management for them. (39)

Although we are still a long way from a full understanding about the impact of genetics on pain, we do know that an individual's genetic profile can strongly influence the effectiveness of some pain medications. An important example is a gene known as CYP2D6, which codes for an enzyme involved in the breakdown of many medicines.

A bit of background: most medications are modified by the body; i.e., metabolized, before they are excreted. A major way that medications are modified involves a family of enzymes called cytochrome P450 (CYP). There are several different CYP enzymes. One of the CYP enzymes involved in the breakdown of many drugs, including the strong opioids, is CYP2D6. But CYP2D6 exists in multiple forms, which differ in their level of enzymatic activity. An individual's genetic profile determines the types of CYP2D6 enzymes he has and therefore influences the rate at which opioids are broken down in his body. (40)

The importance of the various CYP2D6 forms was highlighted at a recent meeting of the American Academy of Pain Medicine. Ramesh Singa reported that one of his patients with severe chronic back and leg pain had been taking escalating doses of oxycodone with no relief. Genetic testing subsequently revealed that this individual had forms of CYP2D6 which broke down oxycodone very rapidly, so it was not present in the body long enough to be effective. The patient switched to a different pain medication, which was not broken down by CYP2D6, and obtained substantial pain relief. (41) Approximately 6 in every 100 people, like this individual, have a CYP2D6 genotype that results in very rapid breakdown of some drugs including oxycodone, preventing effective pain relief. Conversely, 3 in every 100 people have a different CYP2D6 profile that breaks down oxycodone very slowly, potentially causing dangerous side effects and even an overdose. (42)

It is a different story with the weaker opioids tramadol and codeine. Both are widely prescribed for moderate pain. Codeine is often combined with acetaminophen in the drug known as *Tylenol #3*™. Both tramadol and codeine are prodrugs, meaning that they must be transformed to the active form before they can relieve pain. Interestingly, CYP2D6 is one of the main enzymes that transforms tramadol and codeine to their active forms. As a result, people with highly active forms of CYP2D6 may obtain pain relief from tramadol or codeine but little relief from oxycodone. (40) Genetic testing can help determine which type of opioid will provide better pain relief for an individual. (41, 42)

The types of CYP2D6 enzymes in an individual vary with ethnic and racial backgrounds. Up to 30% of people from North Africa and the Arab countries have the types of CYP2D6 which metabolize tramadol and codeine rapidly to their active forms. (40) As a result, they may receive rapid pain relief from tramadol and Tylenol™ with codeine. In contrast, approximately 3-10% of Caucasians, 3.5-8% of African Americans and 1% of Asians have CYP2D6 forms which metabolize tramadol and codeine slowly, resulting in little pain relief from these medications. (40, 43-45) So, if you find that tramadol or Tylenol™ with codeine provides little pain relief, it is possible that the reason is your genetic make-up.

Consider the scenario in which a patient tells his physician that tramadol, which the physician had prescribed, does not relieve his pain and therefore he asks for a stronger medication. Since physicians are currently being strongly warned to be on the lookout for drug-seeking behaviors, they may not trust a patient and as a result may not prescribe one of the stronger opioids. Genetic testing could determine whether the patient's CYP enzymes do not efficiently convert tramadol to its active form. The testing results could then assist the physician in deciding whether to prescribe a strong opioid for this patient. (44)

Other genes besides CYP2D6 are also involved in metabolizing many medications, including those for relieving pain. One of these other genes is CYP2C19, which like CYP2D6 has a variety of forms, resulting in a spectrum of individuals ranging from ultra-rapid to poor metabolizers of certain drugs. The combination of the types of CYP2D6 and CYP2C19 which an individual possesses can significantly influence a person's response to certain medications. A guideline recently provided recommendations about the use and dose of tricyclic antidepressants for managing neuropathic pain in individuals who had varying forms of CYP2D6 and CYP2C19. (46)

Several companies now provide genetic testing for CYP2D6 and other enzymes that break down medications. CYP2D6 genotyping is currently covered by most private insurers and in some cases by Medicare. Genotyping is being used in some academic medical centers to help guide physicians in prescribing medications for their patients, but this is seldom done in private practice. (47) Perhaps in the future, genotyping of each individual will be performed and the data made available, so that health care providers can more accurately determine whether an individual will respond to a given pain medication.

CONCLUSION: THERE IS HOPE FOR THE FUTURE!

Although existing pain medications can effectively relieve minor aches and pains, they are not risk-free and most have only modest, if any, effects on more severe pain. Opioids are the only current medications that relieve severe pain, but they are easily and frequently abused. Better pain medications or alternative pain-relieving methods are greatly needed. Unfortunately, recent increased knowledge about pain has not yet yielded dramatic breakthroughs in new pain treatments which are low risk, affordable and do not require invasive methods such as surgery. Nevertheless, ongoing pain research in academia, biotech companies, and the pharmaceutical industry is continuing to provide new insights into the complexities of pain. Perhaps it is only a matter of time before new medications or alternative methods are discovered that are as effective, either alone or in combination, as the opioids in relieving severe pain but do not have the risks of abuse or addiction. In the meantime, it is important to recognize that prescription opioids are still the most effective medications to relieve many types of severe pain and that the benefits outweigh the risks for many people.

Chapter 7 discussed that opioid abuse has led to increased prescribing regulations. As a result, a new problem has emerged. People who had been using strong opioids for years to relieve their severe chronic pain now often find that their physicians will no longer prescribe the medications they need. The problem is especially difficult when a pain clinic or a pharmacy has been shut down with little notice due to illegal operations. However, the US Justice Department is reportedly working with local agencies to help affected patients find an appropriate physician and pharmacy. (48) On the local level, the health department in the state of Tennessee is proactively contacting patients, helping them find a physician and pharmacy so they can continue to obtain prescription opioids. (48)

Greater access to treatment for addiction and increased availability of the opioid antagonist naloxone are expected to reduce the number of tragic deaths from opioid overdoses. There are signs that the US government and regulatory agencies are beginning to take more realistic and compassionate views about opioid abuse. Some of these were discussed in Chapter 7. There are other encouraging signs. In 2016, the former US Surgeon General Vivek Murthy issued a significant report calling for a cultural shift in our views about addiction. He stated that addiction is not a moral failing; it is a chronic disease which should be viewed with compassion and effectively treated. (49) Also in 2016, the US Food and Drug Administration (FDA) stated that the current opioid abuse crisis is a public health issue, not simply a regulatory issue. (50) The FDA called for expanded development and use of opioid formulations with less potential for abuse, increased access to medications which reverse opioid overdoses, and continued research to discover and develop new non-opioid medications to effectively alleviate moderate to severe pain. (50)

Unfortunately, the US federal government reported in March 2019 that over 80% of the ~2 million people in the US who suffer from opioid addiction are *still* not getting medications to treat their addiction. (51, 52) As stated in a *New York Times* editorial describing the government's report, "This denial of care is so pervasive and egregious.... that it amounts to a serious ethical breach on the part of both health care providers and the criminal justice system." (51) The National Academies of Sciences issued a report in 2019, calling for removal of the barriers that limit access to medication-assisted treatment. As discussed in Chapter 7, the report emphasized that opioid addiction is a disease, just as hypertension and diabetes are diseases which can be effectively managed through medications. (52) Certainly there are encouraging signs that governmental agencies are slowly moving away from a purely criminalization model about drug abuse to one that provides help to individuals suffering from the disease of opioid addiction. Hopefully such initiatives will continue to expand so that appropriate treatments for opioid abuse become widely available to all who need it.

In addition to the ongoing opioid abuse problem, the problem of unrelieved pain is still very much with us. Although pain is personal and "is what the patient says it is," there is a real need for objective measures of pain. Such objective measures would assist in improving pain relief, especially for patients with chronic pain when an obvious cause of the pain could not be found. Objective measures of pain would help physicians determine appropriate treatments. In addition, objective pain measurement would remove much of the concern by physicians that patients may be fabricating their pain for the purpose of obtaining drugs or supporting dubious disability claims. Advances in imaging technologies may yield new methodologies which will enable objective determination of pain, without relying solely on the patient's self-report.

Perhaps in the future, personalized medicine will become feasible for pain relief. Brain imaging and genetics studies may eventually help a clinician select the most appropriate pain-relieving treatment for a particular patient. Due to the overall complexities of pain and individual differences, personalized treatment may be needed to significantly improve pain relief in the future. (53)

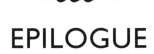

EPILOGUE

In the Introduction, I posed several questions about pain and the suffering caused by unrelieved pain. The chapters that followed attempted to answer these questions, although they probably raised other questions as well.

Perhaps the most basic question is whether unrelieved pain actually is a major problem today. The book presents evidence that unrelieved pain *is* pervasive throughout the world, even in developed countries such as the United States. Moreover, pain relief is not provided equitably, since large racial and age disparities exist.

But, why do so many people continue to suffer from pain in spite of modern advances in medicine? As discussed throughout the book, pain is highly complex, both medically and culturally. The multiple reasons for widespread unrelieved pain constituted a major focus of this book.

One reason is that existing medications and alternative methods either are often poorly effective and/or have significant side effects. Treatment of chronic pain is especially difficult. Although our understanding of pain has certainly increased in recent years, there is still much that we do not understand. Hopefully, ongoing research will provide new insights and will eventually yield more effective, affordable and safer ways to relieve pain. Unfortunately, pain research today is poorly funded, both by the government and by the private sector, in comparison to funding for other human afflictions. Perhaps this book will provide an impetus for more research to address the widespread problem of unrelieved pain.

Another reason for inadequate pain relief is that a person's pain may not be taken seriously by others, including health care providers. There is no objective way for a physician to measure a person's pain, so the level of pain is often underestimated and therefore inadequately treated.

Any contemporary book about pain necessarily includes a discussion of opioids, which currently are the *only* medications that can effectively relieve severe pain for many people. Unfortunately, opioids are easily abused, which has led to the current opioid crisis. There are many causes for the crisis, including pharmaceutical companies that downplayed risks of abuse, poor oversight of the wholesale distribution of prescription opioids, and physicians who overprescribed these powerful drugs. The current opioid abuse crisis has caused "opiophobia," both for patients and their health care providers. Patients are often afraid to take opioids to relieve their pain due to fear of addiction. Health care providers and pharmacists are reluctant to prescribe and dispense opioids for fear of contributing to opioid abuse. But many people *do* take opioids long-term to relieve their pain, without becoming addicted. Some new regulations limiting opioid prescriptions are making it difficult for chronic pain patients to obtain the medications which they have responsibly used for years. In Chapter 7, I have attempted to provide a balanced assessment of the risks and benefits of opioids for pain relief, by acknowledging that prescription opioids do have risks but also by emphasizing the right of people to obtain relief from unrelenting pain.

Although the opioid abuse crisis appears to have started with prescription opioids, it is important to recognize that opioid abuse has changed since the early days of the crisis. In 2019, "street drugs" such as heroin and fentanyl, rather than prescription opioids, are the major source of opioid abuse and deaths from drug overdoses. There are encouraging signs that abuse of prescription opioids is decreasing.

Opioid addiction is a disease, not simply a behavior. The problem of addiction will not be alleviated by viewing people suffering from addiction as criminals. Medical treatments exist for opioid abuse disorder, but they are not widely available to all who need them. I advocate for greater access to treatment for those suffering from opioid addiction. In my view, the root of opioid abuse is not the drugs themselves, but rather sociological and economic conditions which give rise to a sense of hopelessness and despair. But this is a different topic for other authors and policymakers to address.

I argue that cultural and religious attitudes about pain also play a significant role in the ongoing suffering from unrelieved pain. The meaning of pain and the importance of pain relief have been controversial through much of human history. Since pain is a subjective experience which can't be truly understood by another person, it has often been misunderstood. Historically, relief of pain has not been considered very important. Christianity, in particular, taught that pain could be a punishment or a blessing, and therefore should simply be endured. Even with medical advances in the 19th and early 20th centuries, the new methodologies which could prevent and relieve pain were not always utilized due to long-standing beliefs and biases.

Although pain does not have religious implications for most people today, the concept that pain has positive aspects still exists. I recently saw a young man wearing a t-shirt that stated: "Pain is weakness leaving the body." This statement is attributed to General Lewis B. Puller of the Marine Corps and is still used as a slogan for recruitment by the Marines. Of course, this statement as used by the Marine Corps emphasizes the value of physical exertion and the need to expend extra effort to enable greater achievement. Nevertheless, when interpreted literally, this statement would imply that pain itself is beneficial.

The historical idea continues that people in pain should simply "buck up." This idea is often part of the modern male ethos. An example is the response to the 2019 retirement of star football quarterback Andrew Luck at age twenty-nine due to pain from multiple football injuries. Many football players and other men were overwhelming negative, saying that as a man he should simply endure the pain and continue his career.

The problem of unrelieved pain is still real and pervasive today. Both cultural views and the limits of medicine contribute to ongoing suffering from pain. Although the importance of pain relief *did* gain attention in the latter part of the 20th century, it is again being devalued today, at least in part because of opioid abuse.

I wrote this book due to my research experience devoted to the discovery of new ways to relieve pain, as well as my firm belief that human suffering should be reduced whenever possible. I sincerely hope that any insight gained from reading this book will contribute to more effective and humane treatment of the many people suffering from unrelieved pain. Finally, I would point out that the book reflects existing scientific understanding, as well as current medical practice, related to pain relief. But this is hardly the last word, since science continues to explore the complexities of pain and pain relief. Moreover, policies about pain management and treatment of opioid addiction will likely undergo changes in the future. I encourage you, dear reader, to follow new developments and to advocate for those who suffer from unrelieved pain, as well as those who suffer from the disease of addiction.

ACKNOWLEDGMENTS

First and foremost, I thank my husband Robert, who provided critical feedback on multiple early versions of the manuscript. I can't adequately express my gratitude for his ongoing support when the task seemed over-whelming. Without his encouragement, this book would never have been completed.

I thank Prisca Honore PhD, Maria Teresa Poblet RN, Douglas Carlson DVM, Carmela Miglionico MHA, and Joyce Palazzotto PhD, who provided helpful comments on various chapters. I also sincerely thank Rudy Shur of Square One Publishers. Although ultimately Square One was not the right fit for publication of this book, Mr. Shur provided extraordinarily helpful recommendations on structure and content of the book. Finally, I thank Outskirts Press for their guidance and commitment to bringing this book to fruition.

ABBREVIATIONS

AAFP: American Academy of Family Physicians
AAP: American Academy of Pediatrics
ACT: Acceptance and Commitment Therapy
AMA: American Medical Association
Anti-NGF mAbs: Monoclonal Antibodies to Nerve Growth Factor
CB1: Cannabinoid Receptor 1
CB2: Cannabinoid receptor 2
CBT: Cognitive Behavioral Therapy
CDC: United States Centers for Disease Control and Prevention
CGRP: Calcitonin Gene-Related Peptide
cLBP: Chronic Low Back Pain
CMS: Centers for Medicare and Medicaid Services
CNS: Central Nervous System
COX: Cyclooxygenase
CV: Cardiovascular
CYP: Cytochrome P450

DEA: Drug Enforcement Agency
ED: Emergency Department
EKG: Electrocardiogram
FDA: United States Federal Drug Administration
FM: Fibromyalgia
fMRI: Functional Magnetic Resonance Imaging
GI: Gastrointestinal
GOPI: Global Opioid Policy Initiative
ICU: Intensive Care Unit
MBSTR: Mindfulness-Based Stress Reduction
MRI: Magnetic Resonance Imaging
MVPA: Multivariate Pattern Analysis
NGF: Nerve Growth Factor
NIH: United States National Institutes of Health
NPS: Neurological Pain Signature
NSAIDs: Non-Steroidal Anti-Inflammatory Drugs
OA: Osteoarthritis
PAG: Periaqueductal Grey
PCA: Patient-Controlled Analgesia
QST: Quantitative Sensory Testing
rTMS: Repetitive Transcranial Magnetic Stimulation
tCDS: Transcranial Direct-Current Stimulation
TENS: Transcutaneous Electrical Stimulation
THC: δ-9-Tetrahydrocannabinol
TRPV1: Transient Receptor Potential Vanilloid 1
US: United States
VA: United States Veteran's Administration
VAS: Visual Analog Scale
WHO: World Health Organization

REFERENCES

Chapter 1.

1. *Bonica's Management of Pain.* Loeser JD, Butler SH, Chapman CR *et al.* (eds.) 3rd Edition. Lippincott, Williams and Wilkins. Philadelphia (2001)
2. *Wall and Melzack's Textbook of Pain.* McMahon SB and Koltzenburg M (eds.) 5th Edition. Elsevier/Churchill Livingstone. Philadelphia (2006)
3. Cox JJ, Reimann F, Nicholas AK, *et al.* An *SCN9A* Channelopathy Causes Congenital Inability to Experience Pain. *Nature* 444:894-898 (2006)
4. Indo Y. Molecular Basis of Congenital Insensitivity to Pain with Anhidrosis (CIPA): Mutations and Polymorphisms in *TRKA (NTRK1)* Gene Encoding the Receptor Tyrosine Kinase for Nerve Growth Factor. *Human Mutation* 18:462-471 (2001)
5. https://migraineresearchfoundation.org/about-migraine/migraine-facts/
6. Mason BN and Russo AF. Vascular Contributions to Migraine: Time to Revisit? *Frontiers in Cellular Neuroscience* 12:233-251(2018) https://doi.org/10.3389/fncel.2018.00233
7. Staud R and Rodriguez ME. Mechanisms of Disease: Pain in Fibromyalgia Syndrome. *Nature Clinical Practice Rheumatology* 2:90-98 (2006)
8. Raffaeli W and Arnaudo E. Pain as a Disease: An Overview. *Journal of Pain Research* 10:2003-2008 (2017)

9. Staud R. Evidence for Shared Pain Mechanisms in Osteoarthritis, Low Back Pain and Fibromyalgia. *Current Rheumatology Reports* 13:513-520 (2011)

10. Julien N, Goffaux P, Arsenault P and Marchand S. Widespread Pain in Fibromyalgia is Related to a Deficit of Endogenous Pain Inhibition. *Pain* 114:295-302 (2005)

11. Jensen KB, Kosek E, Petzke F, *et al*. Evidence of Dysfunctional Pain Inhibition in Fibromyalgia Reflected in rACC During Provoked Pain. *Pain* 144:95-100 (2009)

12. Goffaux P, de Souza JB, Potvin S, and Marchand S. Pain Relief Through Expectation Supersedes Descending Inhibitory Deficits in Fibromyalgia Patients. *Pain* 145:18-23 (2009)

13. Tracey I. Taking the Narrative Out of Pain: Objectifying Pain Through Brain Imaging. Chapter 9. pp. 127-163. In *Narrative, Pain and Suffering*. Carr DB, Loeser JD and Morris DB (eds.) IASP Press. Seattle WA (2005)

14. Catania PN. PCA: Why Is It Popular? *Pain Practitioner* 1:5 (1989)

15. Momeni M, Crucitti M, and De Kock M. Patient-Controlled Analgesia in the Management of Postoperative Pain. *Drugs* 66:2321-2337 (2006)

16. Kong B and Ya Deau JT. Patient-Controlled Analgesia. Chapter 29. pp. 212-216. In *Essentials of Pain Medicine*. 3rd edition (2011)

17. Cervero F. I Feel Your Pain: Perception and the Brain. Chapter 6. pp. 85-98. In *Understanding Pain*. The MIT Press. Cambridge, MA; London, England. (2012)

18. Price DD. Psychological and Neural Mechanisms of the Affective Dimension of Pain. *Science* 288:1769-1772 (2000)

Chapter 2.

1. Dallenbach KM. Pain: History and Present Status. *American Journal of Psychology* 52:331-347 (1939)

2. Linton JJ. *Understanding Pain for Better Clinical Practice. A Psychological Perspective.* Elsevier. Edinburgh; New York (2005)

3. Mowbray D. *Pain and Suffering in Medieval Theology: Academic Debates at the University of Paris in the Thirteenth Century.* p.16. Boydell Press. Woodbridge, Suffolk; Rochester, NY (2009)

4. Dormandy T. Pain Ignored. Chapter 5. pp. 41-45. In *The Worst of Evils: The Fight Against Pain*. Yale University Press. New Haven (2006)

5. Marcus Aurelius Antonius. *Meditations*. Translated and edited by Farquharson, ASL. Book VIII, paragraph #47. Knopf. New York (1946, reprinted 1992)

6. Marcus Aurelius Antonius. *Meditations*. Translated and edited by Farquharson, ASL. Book IX, paragraph #1. Knopf. New York (1946, reprinted 1992)

7. Rey R. *The History of Pain*. Translated by Wallace LE, Cadden JA and Cadden SW. p28. Harvard University Press. Cambridge, MA (1993)

8. Rey R. *The History of Pain*. Translated by Wallace LE, Cadden JA and Cadden SW. pp. 41-43. Harvard University Press. Cambridge, MA (1993)

9. Booth M. *Opium: A History*. St. Martin's Press. New York (1998)

10. Loeser JD. Opiophobia and Opiophilia. pp. 1-4. In *Opioids and Pain Relief: A Historical Perspective*. Meldrum ML (ed) IASP Press. Seattle, WA (2003)

11. Perkins J. *The Suffering Self: Pain and Narrative Representation in the Early Christian Era*. Routledge. London; New York (1995)

12. Dormandy T. Pain Denied. Chapter 4. pp. 34-40. In *The Worst of Evils: The Fight Against Pain*. Yale University Press. New Haven (2006)

13. Cohen E. *The Modulated Scream: Pain in Late Medieval Culture*. pp. 208-211. University of Chicago Press. Chicago; London (2010)

14. Wolterstorff N. The Place of Pain in the Space of Good and Evil. Chapter 14. pp. 406-419. In *Pain and Its Transformations*: *The Interface of Biology and Culture*. Coakley S and Kaufman Shelemay K (eds.) Harvard University Press. Cambridge, MA (2007)

15. Augustine. *The City of God Against the Pagans*. Translated and edited by Dyson RW. Cambridge University Press. Cambridge; New York (1998)

16. Cohen E. *The Modulated Scream: Pain in Late Medieval Culture*. pp. 116-117. University of Chicago Press. Chicago; London (2010)

17. Cohen E. *The Modulated Scream: Pain in Late Medieval Culture*. p. 49. University of Chicago Press. Chicago; London (2010)

18. Cohen E. *The Modulated Scream: Pain in Late Medieval Culture*. p. 34. University of Chicago Press. Chicago; London (2010)

19. Cohen E. *The Modulated Scream: Pain in Late Medieval Culture*. pp. 36 and 189. University of Chicago Press. Chicago; London (2010)

20. Mowbray D. *Pain and Suffering in Medieval Theology: Academic Debates at the University of Paris in the Thirteenth Century*. p.73. Boydell Press. Woodbridge, Suffolk; Rochester NY (2009)

21. Cohen E. *The Modulated Scream: Pain in Late Medieval Culture*. p. 50. University of Chicago Press. Chicago; London (2010)

22. Cohen E. Alleviating Pain. Chapter 3. pp. 87-112. In *The Modulated Scream: Pain in Late Medieval Culture*. University of Chicago Press. Chicago; London (2010)

23. Teresa of Avila. *The Way of Perfection.* Edited and translated by Peers EA. Dover Publication. Mineola, NY (2012)

24. Coakley S. Palliative or Intensification? Pain and Christian Contemplation in the Spirituality of the Sixteenth Century Carmelites. Chapter 5. pp. 77-100. In *Pain and Its Transformations: The Interface of Biology and Culture.* Coakley S and Kaufman Shelemay K. (eds.) Harvard University Press. Cambridge, MA (2007)

25. Berbara M. "Esta pena tan Sabrosa." Teresa of Avila and the Figurative Arts in Early Modern Europe. pp. 267-298. In *The Sense of Suffering: Constructions of Physical Pain in Early Modern Culture.* Van Dijkhuizen JF and Enenkel KAE (eds.) Koninklijke Brill NW. Leiden, the Netherlands (2009)

26. Dormandy T. Foundations. Chapter 13. pp. 111-123. In *The Worst of Evils: The Fight Against Pain.* Yale University Press. New Haven (2006)

27. Van Dijkhuizen JF and Enenkel KAE. Introduction. pp. 1-17. In *The Sense of Suffering: Constructions of Physical Pain in Early Modern Culture.* Van Dijkhuizen JF and Enenkel KAE (eds.) Koninklijke Brill NW. Leiden, the Netherlands (2009)

28. Dormandy T. Heavenly Dreams. Chapter 14. pp. 124-136. In *The Worst of Evils: The Fight Against Pain.* Yale University Press. New Haven (2006)

29. Rey R. *The History of Pain.* Translated by Wallace LE, Cadden JA and Cadden SW. p.83. Harvard University Press. Cambridge, MA (1993)

30. Sydenham T. *The Works of Thomas Sydenham.* Translated from the Latin edition of WA Greenhill, with a life of the author by RG Latham. p. 173. Printed for the Sydenham Society. London (1848-1850)

31. Dormandy T. The Age of the Cathedrals. Chapter 9. pp. 73-82. In *The Worst of Evils: The Fight Against Pain.* Yale University Press. New Haven (2006)

32. Rey R. Pain in the Age of the Enlightenment. Chapter 5. pp. 89-131. In *The History of Pain.* Translated by Wallace LE, Cadden JA and Cadden SW. Harvard University Press. Cambridge, MA (1993)

33. Rey R. *The History of Pain.* Translated by Wallace LE, Cadden JA and Cadden SW. Quote from p.106. Harvard University Press. Cambridge, MA (1993)

34. Cohen E. *The Modulated Scream: Pain in Late Medieval Culture.* pp. 168-169. University of Chicago Press. Chicago (2010)

35. Lyons J. *The House of Wisdom: How the Arabs Transformed Western Civilization.* pp. 5, 86, 154-155. Bloomsbury Press. New York; Berlin; London (2009)

36. Dormandy T. Islam. Chapter 8. pp.61-72. In *The Worst of Evils: The Fight Against Pain.* Yale University Press. New Haven (2006)

37. Levenson JD. Response: The Theology of Pain and Suffering in the Jewish Tradition. pp. 126-132. In *Pain and Its Transformations: The Interface of Biology and Culture.* Coakley S and Kaufman Shelemay K. (eds.) Harvard University Press. Cambridge, MA (2007)

38. Levenson JD. *Creation and the Persistence of Evil: The Jewish Drama of Divine Omnipotence.* Princeton University Press. Princeton, NJ (1994)

39. Benbassa E. Suffering as Identity: The Jewish Paradigm. pp. 195-200. In *Religion: Perspectives from the Engelsberg Seminar 2014.* Almquist K and Linklater A. (eds.) Axel and Margaret Ax:son Johnson Foundation. Stockholm (2015)

Chapter 3.

1. Pernick MS. *A Calculus of Suffering: Pain, Professionalism, and Anesthesia in Nineteenth Century America.* p. 56. Columbia University Press. New York (1985)

2. Newman JH. Affliction, a School of Comfort. Sermon 21. pp. 1149-1156. In *Parochial and Plain Sermons.* Ignatius Press. San Francisco (1997)

3. Newman JH. Endurance, the Christian Portion. Sermon 20. p. 1140. In *Parochial and Plain Sermons.* Ignatius Press. San Francisco (1997)

4. Newman JH. Bodily Suffering. Sermon XI. pp. 168-169. In *John Henry Newman's Selected Sermons.* Ian Ker (ed.) Paulist Press. New York; Mahwah NJ (1994)

5. Rey R. *The History of Pain.* Translated by Wallace LE, Cadden JA and Cadden SW. p 184. Harvard University Press. Cambridge, MA (1993)

6. Curtis HD. *Faith in the Great Physician: Suffering and Divine Healing in American Culture 1860-1900.* p.2 Johns Hopkins University Press. Baltimore (2007)

7. Dormandy T. This Yankee Dodge. Chapter 22. pp. 208-226. In *The Worst of Evils: The Fight Against Pain.* Yale University Press. New Haven (2006)

8. "Anaesthesia" and "Anaesthetics". Text of Oliver Wendell Holmes letter to Dr. Morton. Boston. Nov 21, 1846.

9. Dormandy T. In Gower Street. Chapter 23. pp. 227-230. In *The Worst of Evils: The Fight Against Pain.* Yale University Press. New Haven (2006)

10. Rey R. The 19th Century: The Great Discoveries. Chapter 6. pp. 132-269. In *The History of Pain.* Translated by Wallace LE, Cadden JA and Cadden SW. Harvard University Press. Cambridge, MA (1993)

11. Pernick MS. *A Calculus of Suffering: Pain, Professionalism, and Anesthesia in Nineteenth Century America.* Columbia University Press. New York (1985)

12. Pernick MS. Anesthesia and the Calculus of Suffering: A Critical Evaluation. Chapter 11. pp. 208-239. In *A Calculus of Suffering: Pain, Professionalism, and Anesthesia in Nineteenth Century America.* Columbia University Press. New York (1985)

13. Pernick MS. The Case of McGonigle's Foot: Nonanesthetic Surgery in Postanesthetic America. Chapter 1. pp. 3-8. In *A Calculus of Suffering: Pain, Professionalism, and Anesthesia in Nineteenth Century America.* Columbia University Press. New York (1985)

14. Barry E. Royal Mums Change Birthing Traditions. *New York Times.* May 7, 2019.

15. Pernick MS. The Drawbacks of Anesthesia. Chapter 3. pp. 35-76. In *A Calculus of Suffering: Pain, Professionalism, and Anesthesia in Nineteenth Century America.* Columbia University Press. New York (1985)

16. Bourke J. Religion. Chapter 4. pp. 88-130. In *The Story of Pain: From Prayer to Painkillers.* Oxford University Press. Oxford, UK; New York (2014)

17. Glucklich A. *Sacred Pain: Hurting the Body for the Sake of the Soul.* p. 184. Oxford University Press. Oxford, UK; New York (2001)

18. McGrath PJ and Unruh AM. The History of Pain in Childhood. Chapter 1. pp. 1-43. In *Pain in Children and Adolescents.* Elsevier. Amsterdam; New York (1987)

19. Rey R. *The History of Pain.* Translated by Wallace LE, Cadden JA and Cadden SW. p. 187. Harvard University Press. Cambridge, MA (1993)

20. Flood P. Foreword. In *New Problems in Medical Ethics.* Flood P. (ed.) Translated from the French by Carroll MG. The Mercier Press Ltd. Cork, Ireland (1957)

21. Rey R. *The History of Pain.* Translated by Wallace LE, Cadden JA and Cadden SW. p. 189. Harvard University Press. Cambridge, MA (1993)

22. Dabney RL. *Life of Lieut.-Gen. Thomas J Jackson (Stonewall Jackson)* Vol 2. Chalmers W. (ed.) James Nisbet and Co. London (1866)

23. Rankin M. *The Daughter of Affliction: A Memoir of the Protracted Sufferings and Religious Experiences of Miss Mary Rankin.* 2nd ed. United Brethren Printing Establishment. Dayton, Ohio (1858)

24. Curtis HD. *Faith in the Great Physician: Suffering and Divine Healing in American Culture 1860-1900.* Johns Hopkins University Press. Baltimore (2007)

25. Curtis HD. *Faith in the Great Physician: Suffering and Divine Healing in American Culture 1860-1900*. p. 5. Johns Hopkins University Press. Baltimore (2007)

26. Curtis HD. *Faith in the Great Physician: Suffering and Divine Healing in American Culture 1860-1900*. p. 18. Johns Hopkins University Press. Baltimore (2007)

27. Curtis HD. *Faith in the Great Physician: Suffering and Divine Healing in American Culture 1860-1900*. pp. 24-25. Johns Hopkins University Press. Baltimore (2007)

28. Curtis HD. *Faith in the Great Physician: Suffering and Divine Healing in American Culture 1860-1900*. p. 58. Johns Hopkins University Press. Baltimore (2007)

29. Glover MB. *Science and Health*. Christian Scientist Publishing Company. Boston (1875)

30. Eddy MB. *Science and Health with Key to the Scriptures*. AV Stewart. Boston (1911); First Church of Christ, Scientist. Boston (1994)

31. Osler W. The Faith that Heals. *British Medical Journal* 1:1470 (1910)

32. Allbutt C. Reflections on Faith Healing. *British Medical Journal* 1:1453 (1910)

33. Bourke J. *The Story of Pain. From Prayer to Painkillers*. p. 102. Oxford University Press. Oxford UK; New York (2014)

34. Finney JM. The Significance and Effect of Pain. Ether Day Address Oct 16, 1914 at Massachusetts General Hospital. Quote p. 16. Griffith-Stillings Press. Boston (1914)

35. Gibson PG. Divine Healing. *British Medical Journal* 2:242 (1956)

36. Lewis CS. *The Problem of Pain*. The Macmillan Co. New York (1944)

37. McFadden CJ. The Christian Philosophy of Suffering. Chapter 6. pp. 129-142. In *Medical Ethics*. 2nd ed. FA Davis Company. Philadelphia (1949)

38. Marshall J. *Medicine and Morals*. Vol 129 from the series *20th Century Encyclopedia of Catholicism*. pp. 114-122. Hawthorn Books. New York (1960)

39. Dormandy T. Foundations. Chapter 13. pp. 111-123. In *The Worst of Evils: The Fight Against Pain*. Yale University Press. New Haven (2006)

40. Casselberry WE. Diseases of the Pharynx and Nasopharynx. pp. 415-440. In *An American Text-book of the Diseases of Children*. Starr L (ed.) 2nd edition. W.B. Saunders. Philadelphia (1898)

41. Thorek M. *Modern Surgical Technic*. Vol 3. p. 2021. JB Lippincott Co. Philadelphia (1938)

42. Bourke J. *The Story of Pain. From Prayer to Painkillers*. pp. 275-276. Oxford University Press. Oxford UK; New York (2014)

43. McGrath PJ and Unruh AM. *Pain in Children and Adolescents*. p 27. Elsevier. Amsterdam; New York (1987)

44. Swafford LI and Allan D. Pain Relief in the Pediatric Patient. *Medical Clinics of North America*. 52:131-136 (1968)

45. Eland JM and Anderson JE. The Experience of Pain in Children. pp. 453-476. In *Pain: A Sourcebook for Nurses and Other Health Professionals*. Jacox AK (ed.) Little, Brown and Company. Boston (1977).

46. Beyer JE, DeGood DE, Ashley LC and Russell GA. Patterns of Post-Operative Analgesia Use with Adults and Children Following Cardiac Surgery. *Pain* 17: 71-81 (1983)

47. Walco GA, Cassidy RC and Schechter NL. Pain, Hurt, and Harm--The Ethics of Pain Control in Infants and Children. *New England Journal of Medicine* 331:541-544 (1994)

48. Cunningham N. Chapter 9. Moral and Ethical Issues in Clinical Practice. pp. 255-273. In *Pain in Neonates*. Anand KJS and McGrath PJ (eds.) Elsevier. Amsterdam; New York (1993)

49. Fitzgerald M and Anand KJS. Developmental Neuroanatomy and Neurophysiology of Pain. Chapter 2. pp. 11-31. In *Pain in Infants, Children, and Adolescents*. Schechter NL, Berde CB and Yaster M (eds.) Williams and Wilkins. Baltimore (1993)

50. Schechter NL, Berde CB and Yaster M. Pain in Infants, Children and Adolescents: An Overview. Chapter 1. pp. 3-9. In *Pain in Infants, Children, and Adolescents*. Schechter NL, Berde CB and Yaster M (eds.) Williams and Wilkins. Baltimore (1993)

51. Schechter NL and Allen DA. Physicians' Attitudes toward Pain in Children. *Journal of Developmental and Behavioral Pediatrics* 7:350-354 (1986)

52. Nelson WE. *Textbook of Pediatrics*. WB Saunders Co. Philadelphia (1964)

53. Barnett HL. *Pediatrics*. Appleton-Century-Crofts. New York (1972)

54. Rana SR. Pain – A Subject Ignored. *Pediatrics* 79:309-310 (1987)

55. Rovner S. Surgery Without Anesthesia: Can Preemies Feel Pain? *Washington Post*. August 13, 1986.

56. McGrath PJ and Unruh AM. Social and Legal Issues. Chapter 11. pp. 295-320. In *Pain in Neonates*. Anand KJS and McGrath PJ (eds.) Elsevier. Amsterdam; New York (1993)

57. Koblin DD and Lawson JR. Hyperventilation and Anesthetic Requirement in Babies. *Lancet* 330:1033 (1987)

58. Lawson JR. Pain in the Neonate and Fetus. *New England Journal of Medicine* 318:1398 (1988)

59. Fitzgerald M, Millard C, McIntosh N. Cutaneous Hypersensitivity Following Peripheral Tissue Damage in Newborn Infants and Its Reversal with Topical Anaesthesia. *Pain* 39:31-36 (1989)

60. Anand KJS and Carr DB. The Neuroanatomy, Neurophysiology and Neurochemistry of Pain, Stress, and Analgesia in Newborns and Children. *Pediatric Clinics North America* 36:795-822 (1989)

61. Slater R, Cantarella A, Gallella S, *et al*. Cortical Pain Responses in Human Infants. *Journal of Neuroscience* 26:3662-3666 (2006)

62. Anand KJS. Hormonal and Metabolic Functions of Neonates and Infants Undergoing Surgery. *Current Opinion in Cardiology* 1:681-689 (1986)

63. Forfar JO and Campbell AGM. Medicine and the Media. *British Medical Journal* 295:659-660 (1987)

64. Porter FL, Grunau RE, Anand KJS. Long Term Effects of Pain in Infants. *Journal of Developmental and Behavioral Pediatrics.* 20:253-261 (1999)

65. AAP Committee on Fetus and Newborn and Section on Anesthesiology and Pain Medicine. Prevention and Management of Procedural Pain in the Neonate: An Update. *Pediatrics* 137 (2) e20154271 (2016)

66. Taddio A, Shah V, Gilbert-MacLeod C, and Katz J. Conditioning and Hyperalgesia in Newborns Exposed to Repeated Heel Lances. *Journal of the American Medical Association* 288:857-861 (2002)

67. Taddio A, Katz J, Ilersich AL, and Koren G. Effect of Neonatal Circumcision on Pain Response During Subsequent Routine Vaccination. *Lancet* 349:599-603 (1997)

68. McIlroy L. Forward. pp. 3-4. In *Anaesthesia and Analgesia in Labour*. Lloyd-Williams, KG. W. Wood and Co. Baltimore (1934)

69. Mitchell SW. *Doctor and Patient.* 4th edition. JB Lippincott Co. Philadelphia (1904)

70. Mitchell SW. *Doctor and Patient.* 4th edition. p. 92. JB Lippincott Co. Philadelphia (1904)

71. Macht DI. The History of Opium and Some of its Preparations and Alkaloids. *Journal of the American Medical Association* LXIV: 477-481 (1915)

72. Cowen DL and Helfand WH. *Pharmacy: An Illustrated History.* p. 184. Harry N Abrams Inc. New York (1990)

73. Acker CJ. Take as Directed: The Dilemmas of Regulating Addictive Analgesics and Other Psychoactive Drugs. Chapter 4. p. 38. In *Opioids and Pain Relief: A Historical Perspective*. Meldrum ML. (ed.) IASP Press (2003)

74. Hoyle C. The Care of the Dying. *Post-Graduate Medical Journal*. pp. 119-123. April 1944.

75. Clark D. The Rise and Demise of the Brompton Cocktail. Chapter 6. pp. 85-98. In *Opioids and Pain Relief: A Historical Perspective*. Meldrum ML. (ed.) IASP Press. Seattle (2003)

76. McCaffery M. *Nursing Management of the Patient with Pain*. JB Lippincott Co. Philadelphia (1972)

77. Merriman A. *Audacity to Love: The Story of Hospice Africa: Bringing Hope and Peace for the Dying*. Irish Hospice Foundation. Dublin (2010)

78. Saunders, CM. *Cicely Saunders: Founder of the Hospice Movement: Selected letters 1959-1999*. Clark D. (ed.) Oxford University Press. Clarendon; New York (2002)

79. Bichell RE. How Uganda Came to Earn High Marks for Quality of Death. National Public Radio. January 3, 2016.

Chapter 4.

1. Rey R. *The History of Pain*. Translated by Wallace LE, Cadden JA and Cadden SW. p. 78. Harvard University Press. Cambridge MA (1993)

2. Lewis CS. *The Problem of Pain*. The Macmillan Company. New York (1944)

3. Livingston A. Pain and Analgesia in Domestic Animals. pp. 159-189. In *Comparative and Veterinary Pharmacology*. Cunningham F, Elliott J, Lees P (eds.) Volume 199 of the *Handbook of Experimental Pharmacology*. Springer. Heidelberg; London; New York (2010)

4. McKune CM, Murrell JC, Nolan AM *et al*. Nociception and Pain. Chapter 29. pp. 584-623. In *Veterinary Anesthesia and Analgesia*. Grimm KA, Lamont LA, Tranquilli WJ, Greene SA and Robertson SA. (eds.) Wiley Blackwell. Ames, Iowa (2015)

5. Cadiot PJ and Almy J. *A Treatise on Surgical Therapeutics of Domestic Animals*. Translated by Liautard A. Vol 1 part 2 (1900) and Vol 1 part 3 (1902) WR Jenkins. New York.

6. Liautard A. *A Manual of Operative Veterinary Surgery*. WR Jenkins. New York (1906)

7. Lacroix JV. Castration of Dogs and Cats. pp. 83-86. In *Animal Castration*. American Journal of Veterinary Medicine. (1915)

8. Frank ER. *Veterinary Surgery*. Burgess Publishing Company. Minneapolis (1953)

9. Tranquilli WJ and Grimm KA. Introduction: Use, Definitions, History Concepts, Classification and Considerations for Anesthesia and Analgesia. Chapter 1. pp. 3-10. In *Veterinary Anesthesia and Analgesia*. Grimm KA, Lamont LA, Tranquilli WJ, Greene SA and Robertson SA. (eds.) Wiley Blackwell. Ames, IA (2015)

10. Hancock RCG. *Memoirs of a Veterinary Surgeon*. pp. 172-179. MacGibbon and Kee. London (1952)

11. Stamm GW. *Veterinary Guide for Farmers*. Burch DS. (ed.) Windsor Press. New York (1950)

12. Stamm GW. *Veterinary Guide for Farmers*. Klussendorf RC. (ed.) Hearst Corp. New York (1975)

13. Fradley LF. *The Farm Veterinarian*. CC Thomas. Springfield, IL (1964)

14. Fradley LF. *The Farm Veterinarian*. p. 184. CC Thomas. Springfield, IL (1964)

15. Personal communications. Douglas Carlson DVM, Dennis Carlson, Greg Anderson.

16. McKelvey D and Hollingshead KW. Analgesia. Chapter 8. pp. 315-319. In *Veterinary Anesthesia and Analgesia*. Mosby. St. Louis, MO (2003)

17. Hansen B and Hardie E. Prescription and Use of Analgesics in Dogs and Cats in a Veterinary Teaching Hospital: 258 Cases (1983-1989). *Journal of the American Veterinary Medical Association* 202:1485-1494 (1993)

18. Cadiot PJ and Almy J. *A Treatise on Surgical Therapeutics of Domestic Animals*. Chapter 4. pp. 271-272. Translated by Liautard A. WR Jenkins. New York (1906)

19. Hoskins HR, Lacroix JV and Mayer K. (eds.) *Canine Medicine, A Text and Reference Work*. American Veterinary Publications. Evanston IL (1953)

20. Hoskins HR, Lacroix JV and Mayer K. (eds.) *Canine Medicine, A Text and Reference Work*. p. 135. American Veterinary Publications. Evanston IL (1953)

21. Hoskins HR, Lacroix JV and Mayer K. (eds.) *Canine Medicine, A Text and Reference Work*. p. 89. American Veterinary Publications. Evanston, IL (1953)

22. Honore P, PhD. Personal communication.

23. Hellyer PW. Treatment of Pain in Dogs and Cats. *Journal of the American Veterinary Medical Association* 221:212-215 (2002)

24. *Veterinary Anesthesia and Analgesia*. Grimm KA, Lamont LA, Tranquilli WJ, Greene SA and Robertson SA. (eds.) Wiley Blackwell. Ames, Iowa. (2015)

25. Beswick A, Dewey C, Johnson R, *et al*. Survey of Ontario Veterinarians' Knowledge and Attitudes on Pain in Dogs and Cats in 2012. *Canadian Veterinary Journal* 57:1274-1280 (2016)

26. Stookey JM. The Veterinarian's Role in Controlling Pain in Farm Animals. *Canadian Veterinary Journal* 46:453-456 (2005)

27. Carlson D, DVM. Personal communication.

28. Beston H. *The Outermost House: A Year of Life on the Great Beach of Cape Cod*. Doubleday, Doran and Co., Inc. Garden City, NY (1928)

Chapter 5.

1. Wilson JE and Pendleton JM. Oligoanalgesia in the Emergency Department. *American Journal of Emergency Medicine* 7: 620-623 (1989)

2. Gelinas C. Management of Pain in Cardiac Surgery ICU Patients: Have We Improved Over Time? *Intensive and Critical Care Nursing* 23:298-303 (2007)

3. Jabusch KM, Lewthwaite BJ, Mandzuk LL, *et al*. The Pain Experience of Inpatients in a Teaching Hospital. *Pain Management Nursing* 16:69-76 (2015)

4. Desbiens NA, Wu AW, Broste SK, *et al*. Pain and Satisfaction with Pain Control in Seriously Ill Hospitalized Patients: Findings from the SUPPORT Research Investigations. *Critical Care Medicine* 24: 1953-1961 (1996)

5. Donovan M, Dillon P and McGuire L. Incidence and Characteristics of Pain in a Sample of Medical-Surgical Patients. *Pain* 30:69-78 (1987)

6. Apfelbaum JL, Chen C, Mehta SS, Gan TJ. Postoperative Pain Experience: Results from a National Survey Suggest Postoperative Pain Continues to Be Undermanaged. *Anesthesia and Analgesia* 97:534-540 (2003)

7. Chou R, Gordon DB, de Leon-Casasola OA, *et al*. Management of Postoperative Pain: A Clinical Practice Guideline from the American Pain Society, the American Society of Regional Anesthesia and Pain Medicine, and the American Society of Anesthesiologists' Committee on Regional Anesthesia, Executive Committee, and Administrative Council. *Journal of Pain* 17:131-157 (2016)

8. Joshi GP and Ogunnaike BO. Consequences of Inadequate Postoperative Pain Relief and Chronic Persistent Postoperative Pain. *Anesthesiology Clinics of North America* 23: 21-36 (2005)

9. Kehlet H, Jensen TS, and Woolf CJ. Persistent Postsurgical Pain: Risk Factors and Prevention. *The Lancet* 367: 1618-1625 (2006)

10. van den Beuken-van Everdingen MHJ, de Rijke JM, Kessels AG, *et al.* Prevalence of Pain in Patients with Cancer: A Systematic Review of the Past 40 Years. *Annals of Oncology* 18:1437-1449 (2007)

11. Greco MT, Roberto A, Corli O, *et al.* Quality of Cancer Pain Management: An Update of a Systematic Review of Undertreatment of Patients with Cancer. *Journal of Clinical Oncology* 32:4149-4154 (2014)

12. Ziegler L, Mulvey M, Blenkinsopp A, *et al.* Opioid Prescribing for Patients with Cancer in the Last Year of Life: A Longitudinal Population Cohort Study. *Pain* 157:2445-2451 (2016)

13. Scott-Warren J and Bhaskar A. Cancer Pain Management – Part I: General Principles. *Continuing Education in Anaesthesia, Critical Care and Pain* 14: 278-284 (2014)

14. Von Roenn JH, Cleeland CS, Gonin R, *et al.* Physician Attitudes and Practice in Cancer Pain Management. A Survey from the Eastern Cooperative Oncology Group. *Annals of Internal Medicine* 119:121-126 (1993)

15. "Please, Do Not Make Us Suffer Any More..." Access to Pain Treatment as a Human Right. *Human Rights Watch*. New York (2009)

16. Breitbart W, Rosenfeld BD, Passik SD, *et al.* The Under-Treatment of Pain in Ambulatory AIDS Patients. *Pain* 65:243-249 (1996)

17. Toblin RL, Quartana PJ, Riviere LA, *et al.* Chronic Pain and Opioid Use in US Soldiers After Combat Deployment. *JAMA Internal Medicine* 174:1400-1401 (2014)

18. Cherny NI, Baselga J, de Conno F, and Radbruch L. Formulary Availability and Regulatory Barriers to Accessibility of Opioids for Cancer Pain in Europe: A Report from the ESMO/EAPC Opioid Policy Inititative. *Annals of Oncology* 21: 615-626 (2010)

19. Seya M-J, Gelders SFAM, Achara OU, *et al.* A First Comparison Between the Consumption of and the Need for Opioid Analgesics at Country, Regional and Global Levels. *Journal of Pain and Palliative Care Pharmacotherapy* 25: 6-18 (2011)

20. Duthey B and Scholten W. Adequacy of Opioid Analgesic Consumption at Country, Global, and Regional Levels in 2010, Its Relationship with Development Level, and Changes Compared with 2006. *Journal of Pain and Symptom Management* 47: 283-297 (2014). Adequate consumption was defined as the *per capita* opioid consumption in the top 20 countries, as defined by the Human Development Index.

21. Knaul FM, Farmer PE, Krakauer EL, *et al*. Alleviating the Access Abyss in Palliative Care and Pain Relief – An Imperative of Universal Health Coverage: The *Lancet* Commission Report. The *Lancet* 391:1391-1454 (2018)

22. Horton R. A Milestone for Palliative Care and Pain Relief. The *Lancet* 391:1338-1339 (2018)

23. Christo and Mazloomdoost . Cancer Pain and Analgesia. *Annals of the New York Academy of Sciences* 1138:278-298 (2008)

24. IASP Classification of Chronic Pain. *Pain* Supplement 3: S1-S226 (1986)

25. Harstall C and Ospina M. How Prevalent is Chronic Pain? *Pain Clinical Updates* 11:1-4 (2003).

26. Tsang A, Von Korff M, Lee S, *et al*. Common Chronic Pain Conditions in Developed and Developing Countries: Gender and Age Differences and Comorbidity with Depression-Anxiety Disorders. *Journal of Pain* 9:883-891 (2008)

27. Dahlhamer J, Lucas J, Zelaya C, *et al*. Prevalence of Chronic Pain and High-Impact Chronic Pain Among Adults – United States, 2016. *Morbidity and Mortality Weekly Report* 67:1001-1006 (2018)

28. Interagency Pain Research Coordinating Committee. National Pain Strategy: A Comprehensive Population Health-Level Strategy for Pain. Washington DC: US Department of Health and Human Services National Institutes of Health (2016)

29. Gaskin DJ and Richard P. The Economic Costs of Pain in the United States. *Journal of Pain* 13:715-724 (2012)

30. Kaye AD, Baluch A, and Scott JT. Pain Management in the Elderly Population: A Review. *The Ochsner Journal* 10: 179-187 (2010)

31. Brennan F, Carr DB and Cousins M. Pain Management: A Fundamental Human Right. *Anesthesia and Analgesia* 105:205-221 (2007)

32. Bernabei R, Gambassi G, Lapane K, *et al*. Management of Pain in Elderly Patients with Cancer. *Journal of the American Medical Association* 279:1877-1882 (1998)

33. Auret K and Schug SA. Under-Utilisation of Opioids in Elderly Patients with Chronic Pain. *Drugs and Aging* 22:641-654 (2005)

34. Sengstaken EA and King SA. The Problems of Pain and Its Detection Among Geriatric Nursing Home Residents. *Journal of the American Geriatric Society* 41:541-544 (1993)

35. Teno JM, Weitzen S, Wetle T and Mor V. Persistent Pain in Nursing Home Residents. *Journal of the American Medical Association* 285:2081(2001)

36. Pimentel CB, Briesacher BA, Gurwitz JH, *et al.* Pain Management in Nursing Home Residents with Cancer. *Journal of the American Geriatric Society* 63:633-641 (2015).

37. Hallenback J. Pain Management in American Nursing Homes – A Long Way to Go. *Journal of the American Geriatric Society* 63:642-643 (2015)

38. Tang NKY and Crane C. Suicidality in Chronic Pain: A Review of the Prevalence, Risk Factors and Psychological Links. *Psychological Medicine* 36:575-586 (2006)

39. Petrosky E, Harpaz R, Fowler KA, *et al.* Chronic Pain among Suicide Decedents, 2003-2014: Findings from the National Violent Death Reporting System. *Annals of Internal Medicine* 169:448-455 (2018)

40. Hoy D, March L, Brooks P, *et al.* The Global Burden of Low Back Pain: Estimates from the Global Burden of Disease 2010 Study. *Annals of Rheumatic Diseases* 73:968-974 (2014)

41. Pritchett JW. Quiz: How Much Do You Know About Mechanical Low Back Pain? *Medscape.* Aug 1, 2016.

42. Wheeler AH. Low Back Pain and Sciatica. *Medscape.* Jan 8, 2013.

43. Kelsey JL and White AA. Epidemiology and Impact of Low Back Pain. *Spine* 5:133-142(1980)

44. Cunningham LS and Kelsey JL. Epidemiology of Musculoskeletal Impairments and Associated Disability. *American Journal of Public Health* 74:574-579 (1984)

45. Baliki MN, Chiavlo DR, Geha PY, *et al.* Chronic pain and the Emotional Brain: Specific Brain Activity Associated with Spontaneous Fluctuations of Intensity of Chronic Back Pain. *Journal of Neuroscience* 26:12165-12173 (2006)

46. Cavanaugh JM and Weinstein JN. Low Back Pain: Epidemiology, Anatomy and Neurophysiology. pp. 441-456. In *Textbook of Pain.* Wall PD and Melzack R (eds.) Churchill Livingstone. Edinburgh (1994)

47. Peat G, McCarney R and Croft P. Knee Pain and Osteoarthritis in Older Adults: A Review of Community Burden and Current Use of Primary Health Care. *Annals of Rheumatic Diseases* 60:91-97 (2001)

48. Hunter DJ and Felson DT. Osteoarthritis. *British Medical Journal* 332:639-642 (2006)

49. Williams DA and Clauw DJ. Understanding Fibromyalgia: Lessons from the Broader Pain Research Community. *Journal of Pain* 10:777-791(2009)

50. Cohen H. Controversies and Challenges in Fibromyalgia: A Review and a Proposal. *Therapeutic Advances in Musculoskeletal Dis*ease 9:115-127 (2017)

51. Arnold LM, Hudson JI, Hess EV, *et al.* Family Study of Fibromyalgia. *Arthritis and Rheumatism* 50:944-952 (2004)

52. Bouhassira D, Lanteri-Minet M, Attal N, *et al.* Prevalence of Chronic Pain with Neuropathic Characteristics in the General Population. *Pain* 136:380-387 (2008)

53. Dieleman JP, Kerklaan J, Huygen FJPM, *et al.* Incidence Rates and Treatment of Neuropathic Pain Conditions in the General Population. *Pain* 137:681-688 (2008)

54. *Bonica's Management of Pain.* 3rd Edition. Loeser JD (ed.), Butler SH, Chapman CR, Turk DC (assoc. eds.) Lippincott, Williams & Wilkins. Philadelphia (2001)

55. Seretny M, Currie GI, Sena ES, *et al.* Incidence, Prevalence, and Predictors of Chemotherapy-Induced Peripheral Neuropathy: A Systematic Review and Meta-Analysis. *Pain* 155:2461-2470 (2014)

56. *Pain in Infants, Children and Adolescents.* Schechter NL, Berde CB, and Yaster M (eds.) Williams and Wilkins. Baltimore (1993)

57. *Pain in Infants, Children and Adolescents.* 2nd Ed. Schechter NL, Berde CB, and Yaster M (eds.) Lippincott, Williams and Wilkins. Philadelphia (2003)

58. Schechter NL, Berde CB and Yaster M. Pain in Infants, Children and Adolescents: An Overview. pp. 1-8. In *Pain in Infants, Children, and Adolescents. 2nd Ed.* Schechter NL, Berde CB and Yaster M (eds.) Lippincott, Williams and Wilkins. Philadelphia (2003)

59. Alexander J and Manno M. Underuse of Analgesia in Very Young Pediatric Patients with Isolated Painful Injuries. *Annals of Emergency Medicine* 41:617-622 (2003)

60. American Academy of Pediatrics and Canadian Paediatric Society. Prevention and Management of Pain in the Neonate: An Update. *Pediatrics* 118:2231-2241 (2006)

61. Simons SHP, van Dijk M, Anand, KS, *et al.* Do We Still Hurt Newborn Babies? A Prospective Study of Procedural Pain and Analgesia in Neonates. *Archives of Pediatric and Adolescent Medicine* 157: 1058-1064 (2003)

62. Anand KJS, Johnston CC, Oberlander TF, *et al.* Analgesia and Local Anesthesia During Invasive Procedures in the Neonate. *Clinical Therapeutics* 27: 844-876 (2005)

63. AAP Committee on Fetus and Newborn and Section on Anesthesiology and Pain Medicine. Prevention and Management of Procedural Pain in the Neonate: An Update. *Pediatrics* 137 (Supplement 2) e20154271 (2016)

64. Harrison D, Larocque C, Bueno M, *et al.* Sweet Solutions to Reduce Procedural pain in Neonates: A Meta-Analysis. *Pediatrics* 139 (1) e20160955 (2017)

65. Thorek M. *Modern Surgical Technique.* Vol 3. p. 2021. JB Lippincott Co. Philadelphia (1938)

66. Probst BD, Lyons E, Leonard D, *et al.* Factors Affecting Emergency Department Assessment and Management of Pain in Children. *Pediatric Emergency Care* 21:298-305 (2005)

67. Habich M and Letizia M. Pediatric Pain Assessment in the Emergency Department: A Nursing Evidence-Based Practice Protocol. *Pediatric Nursing* 41:198-202 (2015)

68. Brudvik C, Moutte S-D, Baste V and Morken T. A Comparison of Pain Assessment by Physicians, Parents and Children in an Outpatient Setting. *Emergency Medicine Journal* 34:138-144 (2017)

69. Birnie KA, Chambers CT, Fernandez CV, *et al.* Hospitalized Children Continue to Report Undertreated and Preventable Pain. *Pain Research and Management* 19:198-204 (2014)

70. Kozlowski LL, Kost-Byerly S, Colantuoni E, *et al.* Pain Prevalence, Intensity, Assessment and Management in a Hospitalized Pediatric Population. *Pain Management Nursing* 15:22-35 (2014)

71. Tamayo-Sarver JH, Hinze SW, Cydulka RK, and Baker DW. Racial and Ethnic Disparities in Emergency Department Analgesic Prescription. *American Journal of Public Health.* 93:2067-2073 (2003)

72. Pletcher MJ, Kertesz SG, Kohn MA, and Gonzales R. Trends in Opioid Prescribing by Race/Ethnicity for Patients Seeking Care in US Emergency Departments. *Journal of the American Medical Association* 299: 70-78 (2008)

73. Meghani SH, Byun E and Gallagher RM. Time to Take Stock: A Meta-Analysis and Systematic Review of Analgesic Treatment Disparities for Pain in the United States. *Pain Medicine* 13: 150-174 (2012)

74. Harrison L. Ethnic Disparities in Pain Rx Persist at Qualified Center. *Medscape.* May 29, 2015.

75. Green CR, Ndao-Brumblay SK, West B, and Washington T. Differences in Prescription Opioid Analgesic Availability: Comparing Minority and White Pharmacies Across Michigan. *Journal of Pain* 6: 689-699 (2005)

76. Morrison RS, Wallenstein S, Natale DK, et al. "We Don't Carry That" – Failure of Pharmacies in Predominantly Nonwhite Neighborhoods to Stock Opioid Analgesics. *New England Journal of Medicine* 342: 1023-1026 (2000)

77. Hausmann LRM, Gao S, Lee ES, and Kwoh CK. Racial Disparities in the Monitoring of Patients on Chronic Opioid Therapy. *Pain* 154:46-52 (2013)

78. Hoffman KM, Trawalter S, Axt JR and Oliver MN. Racial Bias in Pain Assessment and Treatment Recommendations, and False Beliefs About Biological Differences Between Blacks and Whites. *Proceedings of the National Academy of Sciences (USA)* 113:4296-4301 (2016)

79. Lowes R. Drop Pain as the Fifth Vital Sign, AAFP Says. *Medscape.* Sept 22, 2016.

80. Ault A. Many Physicians, Nurses Want Pain Removed as Fifth Vital Sign. *Medscape.* Feb 21, 2017.

81. Ault A. Federal Panel Urges Incentives to Prescribe Opioid Alternatives. *Medscape.* Nov 1, 2017.

82. Lowes R. Will Physicians Get Relief on Medicare's Pain Questions? *Medscape.* July 15, 2016.

83. Seers T, Derry S, Seers K, and Moore RA. Professionals Underestimate Patients' Pain: A Comprehensive Review. *Pain* 159:811-818 (2018)

84. De Ruddere L, Goubert L, Stevens M, *et al.* Discounting Pain in the Absence of Medical Evidence is Explained by Negative Evaluation of the Patient. *Pain* 154:669-676 (2013)

85. Deandrea S, Montanari M, Moja L, and Apolone G. Prevalence of Undertreatment in Cancer Pain. A Review of Published Literature. *Annals of Oncology* 19:1985-1991 (2008)

86. Harle, CA, Bauer SE, Hoang HQ, *et al.* Decision Support for Chronic Pain Care: How Do Primary Care Physicians Decide When to Prescribe Opioids? A Qualitative Study. *BMC Family Practice* 16:48-78 (2015)

87. Hill ML and Craig KD. Detecting Deception in Pain Expressions: The Structure of Genuine and Deceptive Facial Displays. *Pain* 98:135-144 (2002)

88. Mittenberg W, Patton C, Canyock EM, and Condit DC. Base Rates of Malingering and Symptom Exaggeration. *Journal of Clinical and Experimental Neuropsychology* 24:1094-1102 (2002).

89. Schumacher KL, West C, Dodd M, *et al.* Pain Management Autobiographies and Reluctance to Use Opioids for Cancer Pain Management. *Cancer Nursing: An International Journal for Cancer Care* 25:125-133 (2002)

90. Brennan F, Carr DB and Cousins M. Pain Management: A Fundamental Human Right. *Anesthesia and Analgesia* 105:205-221 (2007)

91. Sternbach RA. Survey of Pain in the United States: The Nuprin Pain Report. *Clinical Journal of Pain* 2:49-53 (1986)

92. Blumgarten AS. *A Textbook of Medicine for Students in Schools of Nursing.* The Macmillan Company. New York (1932)

93. Graffam S. *Care of the Surgical Patient: A Textbook for Nurses.* McGraw-Hill. New York (1960)

94. Ferrell B, Vironi R, Grant M, *et al.* Analysis of Pain Content in Nursing Textbooks. *Journal of Pain and Symptom Management* 19:216-228 (2000)

95. Nelson WE (ed.) *Textbook of Pediatrics.* WB Saunders. Philadelphia (1964)

96. Barnett HL (ed.) *Pediatrics.* Appleton-Century-Croft. New York (1972)

97. Eland JM and Anderson JE. The Experience of Pain in Children. pp. 453-476. In *Pain: A Sourcebook for Nurses and Other Health Professionals.* Jacox AK (ed.) Little, Brown and Company. Boston (1977)

98. Mezei L, Murinson BB, and the Johns Hopkins Pain Curriculum Development Team. Pain Education in North American Medical Schools. *Journal of Pain* 12:1199-1208 (2011)

99. https://hopkinsmedicine.org/som/curriculum/jgenes_to_societyhttps://hub/jhu.edu/2018/03/19/teaching-new-doctors-to-treat-pain

100. Anderson P. AMA Pain Management Program Aims to Strike a Balance. *Medscape.* July 11, 2013.

Chapter 6.

1. *Cancer Pain Relief.* World Health Organization. Geneva (1986)

2. Norn S, Permin H, Kruse PR, and Kruse E. From Willow Bark to Acetylsalicylic acid. *Dan Medicinhist Arbog* 37:79-98 (2009)

3. Stone E. An Account of the Success of the Bark of the Willow in the Cure of Agues. *Philosophical Transactions of the Royal Society of London* 53: 195-200 (1763)

4. Aspirin™ – An Unparalleled "Career". https://www.bayer.com/en/news-room-aspirin-story-history.pdfx

5. Sneader W. The Discovery of Aspirin: A Reappraisal. *British Medical Journal* 321:1591-1594 (2000)

6. Lanza FL, Chan FKL and Quigley EMM. Guidelines for Prevention of NSAID-Related Ulcer Complications. *American Journal of Gastroenterology* 104:728-738 (2009)

7. Brooks PM and Day RO. COX-2 Inhibitors. *Medical Journal of Australia.* 173:433-436 (2000)

8. Katz JA. COX-2 Inhibition: What We Learned – A Controversial Update on Safety Data. *Pain Medicine* 14:S18-S22 (2013)

9. Kimmel SE, Berlin JA, Reilly M, *et al*. Patients Exposed to Rofecoxib and Celecoxib Have Different Odds of Nonfatal Myocardial Infarction. *Annals of Internal Medicine* 142:157-164 (2005)

10. Trelle S, Reichenbach S, Wandel S, *et al*. Cardiovascular Safety of Non-Steroidal Anti-Inflammatory Drugs: Network Meta-Analysis. *British Medical Journal* 342:c7086 (2011)

11. Gorczyca P, Manniello M, Pisano M, and Avena-Woods C. NSAIDs: Balancing the Risks and Benefits. *US Pharmacist* 41:24-27 (2016)

12. FDA Drug Safety Communication: FDA Strengthens Warning that Nonaspirin Nonsteroidal Anti-Inflammatory Drugs (NSAIDS) Can Cause Heart Attacks or Strokes. July 9, 2015. https://www.fda.gov/Drugs/DrugSafety/ucm451800.html.

13. Curfman G. FDA Strengthens Warning that NSAIDs Increase Heart Attack and Stroke Risk. *Harvard Health Publishing.* Updated August 22, 2017. https://www.health.harvard.edu

14. Brown T. CV Safety of Celecoxib Similar to Naproxen, Ibuprofen, FDA Panels Say. *Medscape*. April 25, 2018.

15. Kaufman DW, Kelly JP, Battista DR, *et al*. Exceeding the Daily Dosing Limit of Nonsteroidal Anti-Inflammatory Drugs Among Ibuprofen Users. *Pharmacoepidemiology and Drug Safety* 27:322-331 (2018)

16. Rapaport L. Many People Take Dangerously High Amounts of Ibuprofen. *Medscape*. Feb 9, 2018.

17. Graham GG and Scott KF. Mechanism of Action of Paracetamol. *American Journal of Therapeutics* 12:46-55 (2005)

18. Food and Drug Administration. Organ-Specific Warnings: Internal Analgesic, Antipyretic, and Antirheumatic Drug Products for Over-the-Counter Human Use – Labeling for Products that Contain Acetaminophen. Guidance for Industry. November 2015.

19. Pendell D. *Pharmakopoeia* p. 126. North Atlantic Books. Berkeley CA (2010).

20. Rey R. *The History of Pain*. Translated by Wallace LE, Cadden JA and Cadden SW. p 83. Harvard University Press. Cambridge, MA. (1993)

21. Sydenham T. *The Works of Thomas Sydenham, MD*. p. 173 Translated from the Latin edition of WA Greenhill, with a life of the author by RG Latham. London. Printed for the Sydenham Society. (1848-1850)

22. Huxtable RJ and Schwarz SKW. The Isolation of Morphine – First Principles in Science and Ethics. *Molecular Interventions* 1:189-191 (2001)

23. Krishnamurti C and Chakra Rao SSC . The Isolation of Morphine by Serturner. *Indian Journal of Anaesthesia* 60:861-862 (2016)

24. DEA Drug Scheduling. https://www.dea.gov/druginfo/ds.shtml

25. World Health Organization. Ensuring Balance in National Policies on Controlled Substances: Guidance for Availability and Accessibility of Controlled Medicines. Geneva (2011)

26. United Nations Office on Drugs and Crime. Ensuring Availability of Controlled Medications for the Relief of Pain and Preventing Diversion and Abuse. Striking the Right Balance to Achieve the Optimal Public Health Outcome. Discussion paper based on a scientific workshop held January 18-19, 2011. United Nations. New York (2011)

27. Moulin DE, Boulanger A, Clark AJ, *et al*. Pharmacological Management of Chronic Neuropathic Pain: Revised Consensus Statement from the Canadian Pain Society. *Pain Research and Management* 19:328-335 (2014)

28. Thurston MM and Nykamp D. Clinical Management of Neuropathic Low Back and Neck Pain. *US Pharmacist* 41:42-45 (2016)

29. Backonja M and Rowbotham MC. Pharmacological Therapy for Neuropathic Pain. Chapter 68. pp. 1075-1083. In *Wall and Melzack's Textbook of Pain*. McMahon SB, and Koltzenburg M. (eds.) Elsevier/Churchill Livingston. Philadelphia (2006)

30. Finnerup NB, Attal N, Haroutounian S, *et al*. Pharmacotherapy for Neuropathic Pain in Adults: a Systematic Review and Meta-Analysis. *Lancet Neurology* 14:162-173 (2015)

31. Allen CA and Ivester JR, Jr. Ketamine for Pain Management. Side effects & Potential Adverse Events. *Pain Management Nursing* 18:372-377 (2017)

32. Schoevers RA, Chaves TV, Balukova SM, *et al*. Oral Ketamine for the Treatment of Pain and Treatment-Resistant Depression. *British Journal of Psychiatry* 208:108-113 (2016)

33. Stoker M, Katz N, Van J, *et al*. Capsaicin 8% Patch in Painful Diabetic Peripheral Neuropathy: A Randomized, Double-Blind, Placebo-Controlled Study. Abstract #64 at the European Association for the Study of Diabetes, 2015

34. McCall B. Capsaicin Patch Approved in EU for Diabetic Neuropathy Pain. *Medscape*. Sept 21, 2015.

35. Simpson RW and Wlodarczyk JH. Transdermal Buprenorphine Relieves Neuropathic Pain: A Randomized, Double-Blind, Parallel-Group, Placebo-Controlled Trial in Diabetic Peripheral Neuropathic Pain. *Diabetes Care* 39: 1493-1500 (2016)
36. McGivern JG. Ziconotide: A Review of Its Pharmacology and Use in the Treatment of Pain. *Neuropsychiatric Disease and Treatment* 3:69-85 (2007)
37. Mittal SO, Safarpour D, and Jabbari B. Botulinum Toxin Treatment of Neuropathic Pain. *Seminars in Neurology* 36:73-83 (2016)
38. Migraine Research Foundation. Migraine Fact Sheet 2015. https://www.migraineresearchfoundation.org/fact-sheet
39. Mason BN and Russo AF. Vascular Contributions to Migraine: Time to Revisit? *Frontiers in Cellular Neuroscience* 12: 233-251 (2018)
40. Ahn AH and Basbaum AI. Where Do Triptans Act in the Treatment of Migraine? *Pain* 115:1-4 (2005)
41. FDA News Release. FDA Approves Novel Preventive Treatment for Migraine. May 17, 2018.
42. Novartis Press Release. Novartis and Amgen Announce FDA Approval of Aimovig™ (erenumab), a Novel Treatment Developed Specifically for Migraine Prevention. May 17, 2018.
43. Miotto K, Cho AK, Khalil MA, *et al.* Trends in Tramadol: Pharmacology, Metabolism and Misuse. *Anesthesia and Analgesia* 124:44-51 (2017)

Chapter 7.

1. *Wall and Melzack's Textbook of Pain.* McMahon SB and Koltzenburg M (eds.) Elsevier/Churchill Livingston. Philadelphia. (2006)
2. Anderson P. Expert Panel Final Report on Opioids in Chronic Pain. *Medscape.* Jan 13, 2015.
3. Chou R, Turner JA, Devine EB, *et al.* The Effectiveness and Risks of Long-Term Opioid Therapy for Chronic Pain: A Systematic Review for a National Institutes of Health Pathways to Prevention Workshop. *Annals of Internal Medicine* 162: 276-286 (2015)
4. Editorial. Painkiller Abuses and Ignorance. *New York Times.* March 2, 2015.
5. Furlan AD, Chaparro LE, and Irvin E, Mailis-Gagnon A. A Comparison Between Enriched and Nonenriched Enrollment Randomized Withdrawal Trials of Opioids for Chronic Noncancer Pain. *Pain Research and Management* 16:337-351 (2011)

6. Krebs EE, Gravely A, Nugent S, *et al*. Effect of Opioid vs Nonopioid Medications on Pain-Related Function in Patients with Chronic Back Pain or Hip or Knee Osteoarthritis Pain. The SPACE Randomized Clinical Trial. *Journal of the American Medical Society* 319:872-882 (2018)

7. Anderson P. Eliminating Opioids for Chronic Pain Unwise? *Medscape*. Nov 1, 2017.

8. Kroenke K and Cheville A. Management of Chronic Pain in the Aftermath of the Opioid Backlash. *Journal of the American Medical Association* 317:2365-2366 (2017)

9. Lin KW. Limiting Opioid Prescribing: The Fallout from Rules Telling Doctors How to Prescribe. *Medscape*. May 8, 2018.

10. Guskin E. Poll Details How Opioids Affect the Lives of Users. *Washington Post*. Dec 22, 2016.

11. Clement S and Bernstein L. One-Third of Long-Term Users Say They're Hooked on Prescription Opioids. *Washington Post*. Dec 9, 2016.

12. Rudd RA, Seth P, David F, Scholl L. Increases in Drug and Opioid-Involved Overdose Deaths – United States, 2010-2015. *Morbidity and Mortality Weekly Report* 65:1445-1452 (2016)

13. Lowes R. CDC: Painkillers Not Driving Spike in Fatal Opioid Overdoses. *Medscape*. Dec 19, 2016.

14. Katz J. New Count of 2016 Drug Deaths Shows Accelerated Rate. *New York Times*. Sept 3, 2017.

15. Dowell D, Noonan RK, Houry D. Underlying Factors in Drug Overdose Deaths. *Journal of the American Medical Association* 318:2295-2296 (2017)

16. Seth P, Scholl L, Rudd RA, Bacon S. Overdose Deaths Involving Opioids, Cocaine, and Psychostimulants – United States, 2015-2016. *Morbidity and Mortality Weekly Report* 67:349-358 (2018)

17. Jones CM, Einstein EB, Compton WM. Changes in Synthetic Opioid Involvement in Drug Overdose Deaths in the United States, 2010-2016. *Journal of the American Medical Association* 319:1819-1821 (2018)

18. Yasgur BS. Synthetic Opioids Now Most Common Drugs in Overdose Deaths. *Medscape*. May 1, 2018.

19. Kiang MV, Basu S, Chen J and Alexander MJ. Assessment of Changes in the Geographical Distribution of Opioid-Related Mortality Across the United States by Opioid Type, 1999-2016. *JAMA Network Open*. Feb 22, 2019.

20. Compton WM, Jones CM and Baldwin GT. Relationship Between Nonmedical Prescription-Opioid Use and Heroin Use. *New England Journal of Medicine* 374:154-163 (2016)

21. Unick G, Rosenblum D, Mars S and Ciccarone D. The Relationship Between US Heroin Market Dynamics and Heroin-Related Overdose, 1992-2008. *Addiction* 109:1889-1898 (2014)

22. Szalavitz M. Heroin. *Washington Post*. March 6, 2016.

23. Davis AC, Boburg S, and O'Harrow R. Makers of Generics Had Key Role in Drug Crisis, Records Show. *Washington Post*. July 28, 2019.

24. Bernstein L, Fallis DS, and Higham S. How Drugs Intended for Patients Ended Up in the Hands of Illegal Users: 'No One Was Doing Their Job'. *Washington Post*. Oct 22, 2016.

25. Cicero TJ, Ellis MS, and Kasper ZA. Increased Use of Heroin as an Initiating Opioid of Abuse. *Addiction Behaviors* 74:63-66 (2017)

26. Foley KM. Current Controversies in Opioid Therapy. Chapter 1. pp. 3-11. In *Opioid Analgesics in the Management of Clinical Pain.* Foley KM and Inturrisi CE (eds.) Raven Press. New York (1986)

27. Noble M, Treadwell JR, Tregear SJ *et al.* Long-Term Opioid Management for Chronic Noncancer Pain. *Cochrane Database of Systematic Reviews* 1: CD006605 (2010)

28. Editorial. The Opioid Crisis Foretold. *New York Times.* April 22, 2018.

29. Porter J and Jick H. Addiction Rare in Patients Treated with Narcotics. *New England Journal of Medicine* 302:123 (1980)

30. Schulte F. Purdue Pharma's Sales Pitch Downplayed Risks of Opioid Addiction. *Medscape.* Aug 24, 2018.

31. Fishbain DA, Cole B, Lewis J, Rosomoff HL, Rosomoff RS. What Percentage of Chronic Nonmalignant Pain Patients Exposed to Chronic Opioid Analgesic Therapy Develop Abuse/Addiction and/or Aberrant Drug-Related Behaviors? A Structured Evidence-Based Review. *Pain Medicine* 9:444-459 (2008)

32. Ives TJ, Chelminski PR, Hammett-Stabler CA, *et al.* Predictors of Opioid Misuse in Patients with Chronic Pain: A Prospective Cohort Study. *BMC Health Services Research* 6:46-55 (2006).

33. Gardner EL. What We Have Learned About Addiction from Animal Models of Drug Self-Administration. *American Journal on Addictions* 9:285-313 (2000)

34. Webster LR. *The Painful Truth: What Chronic Pain Is Really Like and Why It Matters to Each of Us*. Webster Media LLC. Salt Lake City, Utah (2015)

35. Agrawal A, Verweij KJH, Gillespie NA, *et al*. The Genetics of Addiction – A Translational Perspective. *Translational Psychiatry*. Jul 2(7) e140. doi: 10.1038/tp.2012.54 (2012)

36. Wax-Thibodeaux E. Veterans Grapple with Restrictions on Narcotics. *Washington Post*. Feb 19, 2015.

37. Dowell D, Haegerich TM, and Chou R. CDC Guideline for Prescribing Opioids for Chronic Pain – United States, 2016. *MMWR Recommendations and Reports* 65:1-49 (2016). DOI:http://dx.doi.org/10.15585/mmwr.rr6501e1.

38. Argoff CE. Commentary. New CDC Opioid Guidelines: The Good, the Bad, the Ugly. *Medscape*. May 13, 2016.

39. Cohen B. CDC Opioid Prescribing Guidelines Misguided, Docs Say. *Medscape*. April 8, 2016

40. Demirjian K and Bernstein L. CDC Warns Doctors About Prescribing Opioid Painkillers. *Washington Post*. March 16, 2016.

41. Argoff CE. Commentary. Readers Respond: Stop Stigmatizing Opioids. *Medscape*. July 5, 2018.

42. Hoffman J and Goodnough A. Rule Led to Big Drop in Opioid Prescriptions; Too Big, Some Doctors Say. *New York Times*. March 7, 2019.

43. Lowes R. Express Scripts Limits on Opioids Rankles Physicians. *Medscape*. Aug 22, 2017.

44. Argoff CE. Commentary. Conflating Effective Chronic Pain Management and Opioid Abuse Potential. *Medscape*. April 14, 2017.

45. Lavin RA, Kalia N, Yuspeh L, *et al*. Work-Enabling Opioid Management. *Journal of Occupational and Environmental Medicine* 59: 761-764 (2017)

46. Shepperd JR and Hale SE. Nurse Practitioners in the World of Pain Management. A Cautionary Tale. *Journal for Nurse Practitioners* 12:102-108 (2016)

47. Ault A. Opioid Epidemic Alters Prescriber, Pharmacist Habits. *Medscape*. Nov 2, 2017.

48. Clark C. Doctors Call California's Probe of Opioid Deaths a 'Witch Hunt'. *Medscape*. Jan 30, 2019.

49. Annual Surveillance Report of Drug-Related Risks and Outcomes. Centers for Disease Control and Prevention. (2017)

50. Goodnough A and Tavernise S. Prescription Dip Seen as Advance in Opioid Battle. *New York Times*. May 22, 2016.

51. Emery G. Cutbacks by Some Doctors Halved New Opioid Prescriptions Over 5 Years. *Medscape*. March 20, 2019.

52. Mulcahy N. A Different Kind of Opioid Crisis in Cancer Patients. *Medscape.* Sept 21, 2016.

53. Ault A. Cancer Patients Face Difficulties in Getting Opioids. *Medscape.* June 26, 2018.

54. Comerci G, Katzman J and Duhigg D. Perspective. Controlling the Swing of the Opioid Pendulum. *New England Journal of Medicine* 378:691-693 (2018)

55. Lagisetty PA, Healy N, Garpestad C, *et al.* Access to Primary Care Clinics for Patients With Chronic Pain Receiving Opioids. *JAMA Network Open.* e196928.doi:10.1001 (2019)

56. Manchikanti L, Damron KS, Beyer CD and Pampati V. A Comparative Evaluation of Illicit Drug Use in Patients With or Without Controlled Substance Abuse in Interventional Pain Management. *Pain Physician* 6:281-285 (2003)

57. Cherny NI, Baselga J, de Conno F and Radbruch L. Formulary Availability and Regulatory Barriers to Accessibility of Opioids for Cancer Pain in Europe: A Report from the ESMO/EAPC Opioid Policy Initiative. *Annals of Oncology* 21:615-626 (2010)

58. Brauser D. Opioid Prescriber Monitoring May Increase Overdose Deaths. *Medscape.* Dec 12, 2014.

59. McNeil Jr DG. 'Opiophobia' and Agony. *ScienceTimes. The New York Times.* Dec 5, 2017.

60. Nelson R. 'Tragedy' of Millions of Cancer Patients Not Getting Opioids. *Medscape.* Dec 4, 2013.

61. Opioid Price Watch Project. Published on line by the International Association for Hospice and Palliative Care. http://hospicecare.com/home/

62. Zogenix News Release. Zogenix Receives FDA approval of New Formulation of Zohydro®ER. Jan 30, 2015.

63. Package insert for Zohydro®ER.

64. Anderson P. New Tamper-Proof Pain Products in the Pipeline. *Medscape.* Sept 14, 2015.

65. Anderson P. FDA Okays Morphine Sulfate (Arymo ER) for Chronic Pain. *Medscape.* Jan 10, 2017.

66. Egalet Corporation Newswire. Egalet Announces Positive Top-Line Results from Phase 3 Study Evaluating Efficacy and Safety of Egalet-002 in Patients with Moderate-to-Severe Chronic Low Back Pain. Nov 28, 2017.

67. Pfizer Press Release. FDA Approves Abuse Deterrent Labeling for EMBEDA® (Morphine Sulfate and Naltrexone Hydrochloride) Extended-Release (ER) Capsules. Oct 17, 2014.

68. Taylor R, Raffa RB, and Pergolizzi JV. Opioid Formulations with Sequestered Naltrexone: A Perspective Review. *Therapeutic Advances in Drug Safety* 5:129-137 (2014)

69. Litman RS, Pagan OH, Cicero TJ. Abuse-Deterrent Opioid Formulations. *Anesthesiology* 128: 1015-1026 (2018)

70. Kristof N. A Mass Killer We're Meeting with a Shrug. *New York Times*. June 22, 2017.

71. Kennedy PJ. The Problem Isn't Just Pills. *Washington Post*. Oct 25, 2015.

72. US Senate Hearing: Homeland Security and Governmental Affairs Committee. ROUNDTABLE – America's Insatiable Demand for Drugs: Examining Alternative Approaches. June 15, 2016.

73. Courtwright DT. *Dark Paradise: A History of Opiate Addiction in America.* Harvard University Press. Cambridge, MA (2001)

74. National Public Radio. Desperate Cities Consider 'Safe Injection' Sites for Opioid Users. *Morning Edition*. Jan 10, 2018.

75. Colliver V, Goldberg D, and Roubein R. Trump Administration Warns California Against 'Safe' Opioid Injection Sites. *Politico*. Aug 28, 2018.

76. Vestal C. Even as Opioids Kill Thousands, Most Clinics Spurn a Lifesaving Treatment. *Washington Post*. Jan 19, 2016.

77. Vestal C. In Opioid Crisis, Methadone Clinics See Revival. *Washington Post*. Nov 13, 2018.

78. Melville NA. Buprenorphine 'Underused" in Primary Care as Opioid Abuse Soars. *Medscape*. May 20, 2016.

79. Melville NA. SAMHSA Expands Access to Buprenorphine for Opioid Dependence. *Medscape*. July 7, 2016.

80. AMA Report Shows National Progress Toward Reversing Opioid Epidemic. May 31, 2018. https://www.ama-assn.org/ama-report-shows-national-progress-toward-reversing-opioid-epidemic.

81. Jamison P. Opioid Treatment with Buprenorphine Will Be Offered at 3 Emergency Rooms. *Washington Post*. May 1, 2019.

82. Brooks M. FDA OKs Buprenorphine Implant (*Probuphine*) for Opioid Dependence. *Medscape*. May 26, 2016.

83. Harper J. A Drugmaker Tries to Cash in on the Opioid Epidemic, One State Law at a Time. National Public Radio. *All Things Considered*. June 12, 2017.

84. Kaplan S. F.D.A. to Expand Medication-Assisted Therapy for Opioid Addicts. *New York Times. Feb 25, 2018.*

85. Subcommittee on Labor, Health and Human Services, Education and Related Agencies. Hearing titled "Addressing the Opioid Crisis in America: Prevention, Treatment & Recovery". Dec 5, 2017.

86. Young KD. House Subcommittee Approves Opioid Package. *Medscape*. April 26, 2018.

87. House Committee on Appropriations. FY2018 Omnibus Fighting the Opioid Epidemic. https://appropriations.house.gov/uploadedfiles/03.21.18_fy18_omnibus_-_opioids_-_one_pager.pdf

Chapter 8.

1. Hill KP, Palastro MD, Johnson B, and Ditre JW. Cannabis and Pain: A Clinical Review. *Cannabis and Cannabinoid Research* 2: 96-104 (2017)

2. Whiting PF, Wolff RF, Deshpande S, *et al*. Cannabinoids for Medical Use: A Systematic Review and Meta-analysis. *Journal of the American Medical Association* 313:2456-2473 (2015)

3. Meng H, Johnston B, Englesakis M, *et al*. Selective Cannabinoids for Chronic Neuropathic Pain. A Systematic Review and Meta-analysis. *Anesthesia and Analgesia* 125:1638-1652 (2017)

4. Medical Letter on Drugs and Therapeutics. Cannabis and Cannabinoids. *Journal of the American Medical Association* 316:2424-2425 (2016)

5. https://gwpharma.com . Website of GW Pharmaceuticals which developed Sativex®.

6. Stockings E, Campbell G, Hall WD, *et al*. Cannabis and Cannabinoids for the Treatment of People with Chronic Noncancer Pain Conditions: A Systematic Review and Meta-analysis of Controlled and Observational Studies. *Pain* 159:1932-1954 (2018)

7. Häuser W, Finnerup NB, Moore RA. Systematic Reviews with Meta-analysis on Cannabis-Based Medicines for Chronic Pain: A Methodological and Political Minefield. *Pain* 159:1906-1907 (2018)

8. Pertwee RG. Targeting the Endocannabinoid System with Cannabinoid Receptor Agonists: Pharmacological Strategies and Therapeutic Possibilities. *Philosophical Transactions of the Royal Society of London B Biological Science* 367:3353-3363 (2012)

9. Atwood BK, Straiker A, and Mackie K. CB2: Therapeutic Target-In-Waiting. *Progress in Neuropsychopharmacology and Biological Psychiatry* 38:16-20 (2012)

10. Dhopeshwarkar A and Mackie K. CB2 Cannabinoid Receptors as a Therapeutic Target – What Does the Future Hold? *Molecular Pharmacology* 86:430-437 (2014)

11. Ibrahim MM, Deng H, Zvonok A, *et al*. Activation of CB2 Cannabinoid Receptors by AM1241 Inhibits Experimental Neuropathic Pain: Pain Inhibition by Receptors Not Present in the CNS. *Proceedings of the National Academy of Sciences (USA)* 100:10529-10533 (2003)

12. Arena Pharmaceuticals Website. https://www. arenapharm.com/pipeline. Accessed Feb 22, 2019.

13. Mulpuri Y, Marty VN, Munier JJ, *et al*. Synthetic Peripherally-Restricted Cannabinoid Suppresses Chemotherapy-Induced Peripheral Neuropathy Pain Symptoms by CB1 Receptor Activation. *Neuropharmacology* 139:85-97 (2018)

14. Gado F, Mannelli L DC, Lucarini E, *et al*. Identification of the First Synthetic Allosteric Modulator of the CB2 Receptors and Evidence of its Efficacy for Neuropathic Pain Relief. *Journal of Medicinal Chemistry* 62:276-287 (2019)

15. Stevens R, Hanson P, Wei N, *et al*. Safety and Tolerability of CNTX-4975 in Subjects with Chronic, Moderate to Severe Knee Pain Associated with Osteoarthritis (OA): A Pilot Study. *Journal of Pain* 18: S70 Abstract 382. (2017)

16. https://www.centrexion.com. Centrexion Therapeutics Website. Press Releases: Jan 2, 2018; March 27, 2019; June 11, 2019.

17. Surowy CS, Kym PR and Reilly RM. Biochemical Pharmacology of TRPV1: Molecular Integrator of Pain Signals. Chapter 3. pp. 101-133 In *Vanilloid Receptor TRPV1 in Drug Discovery. Targeting Pain and Other Pathological Disorders.* Gomtsyan A and Faltynek CR (eds.) John Wiley & Sons Inc. Hoboken NJ (2010)

18. Surowy CS, Neelands TR, Bianchi BR, *et al*. (*R*)-(5-*tert*-Butyl-2,3-dihydro-1*H*-inden-1-yl)-3-(1*H*-indazol-4-yl)-urea (ABT-102) Blocks Polymodal Activation of Transient Receptor Potential Vanilloid 1 Receptors *in vitro* and Heat-Evoked

Firing of Spinal Dorsal Horn Neurons *in vivo. Journal of Pharmacology and Experimental Therapeutics* 326:879-888 (2008)

19. Lee Y, Hong S, Cui M, *et al*. Transient Receptor Potential Vanilloid Type 1 Antagonists: A Patent Review (2011-2014). *Expert Opinion on Therapeutic Patents* 25:291-318 (2015)

20. Aghazadeh Tabrizi M, Baraldi PG, Baraldi S, *et al*. Medicinal Chemistry, Pharmacology and Clinical Implications of TRPV1 Receptor Antagonists. *Medicinal Research Reviews* 37:936-983 (2017)

21. Honore P, Wismer CT, Mikusa J, *et al*. A-425619 [1-Isoquinolin-5-yl-3-(4-trifluormethyl-benzyl)-urea], a Novel Transient Receptor Potential Type V1 receptor antagonist, Relieves Pathophysiological Pain Associated with Inflammation and Tissue Injury in Rats. *Journal of Pharmacology and Experimental Therapeutics* 314:410-421 (2005)

22. Honore P, Chandran P, Hernandez G, *et al*. Repeated Dosing of ABT-102, a Potent and Selective TRPV1 Antagonist, Enhances TRPV1-Mediated Analgesic Activity in Rodents, but Attenuates Antagonist-Induced Hyperthermia. *Pain* 142:27-35 (2009)

23. Chizh BA, Priestley T, Rowbotham M and Schaffler K. Predicting Therapeutic Efficacy – Experimental Pain in Human Subjects. *Brain Research Reviews* 60:243-254 (2009)

24. Schaffler K, Reeh P, Duan WR, *et al*. An Oral TRPV1 Antagonist Attenuates Laser Radiant-Heat-Evoked Potentials and Pain Ratings from UV_B-Inflamed and Normal Skin. *British Journal of Clinical Pharmacology* 75: 404-414 (2013)

25. Chizh BA, O'Donnell MB, Napolitano A, *et al*. The Effects of the TRPV1 Antagonist SB-705498 on TRPV1 Receptor-Mediated Activity and Inflammatory Hyperalgesia in Humans. *Pain* 132:132-141 (2007)

26. Kaneko Y and Szallasi A. Transient Receptor Potential (TRP) Channels: A Clinical Perspective. *British Journal of Pharmacology* 171:2474-2507 (2014)

27. Rowbotham MC, Nothaft W, Duan WR, *et al*. Oral and Cutaneous Thermosensory Profile of Selective TRPV1 Inhibition by ABT-102 in a Randomized Healthy Volunteer Trial. *Pain* 152: 1192-1200 (2011)

28. Caterina MJ, Leffler A, Malmberg AB, *et al*. Impaired Nociception and Pain Sensation in Mice Lacking the Capsaicin Receptor. *Science* 288:306-313 (2000)

29. Davis JB, Gray J, Gunthorpe MJ, *et al*. Vanilloid Receptor-1 Is Essential for Inflammatory Thermal Hyperalgesia. *Nature* 405:183-187 (2000)

30. Wickenden AD and Chaplan SR. Editorial. Once Is Not Enough: Improved Efficacy Following Repeated Dosing with a TRPV1 Antagonist. *Pain* 142:5-6 (2009)

31. Kort ME and Kym PR. TRPV1 Antagonists: Clinical Setbacks and Prospects for Future Development. *Progress in Medicinal Chemistry* 51:57-70 (2012)

32. Lehto SG, Tamir T, Deng H, *et al.* Antihyperalgesic Effects of (R,E)-N-(2-hydroxy-2,3-dihydro-1H-inden-4-yl)-3-(2-(piperidin-1-yl)-4-(trifluoromethyl) phenyl)-acrylamide (AMG8562), a Novel Transient Receptor Potential Vanilloid Type 1 Modulator that Does Not Cause Hyperthermia in Rats. *Journal of Pharmacology and Experimental Therapeutics* 326:218-229 (2008)

33. Reilly RM, McDonald HA, Puttfarcken PS, *et al.* Pharmacology of Modality-Specific Transient Receptor Potential Vanilloid-1 Antagonists that Do Not Alter Body Temperature. *Journal of Pharmacology and Experimental Therapeutics* 342:416-428 (2012)

34. Garami A, Pakai E, McDonald HA, *et al.* TRPV1 Antagonists that Cause Hypothermia, Instead of Hyperthermia, in Rodents: Compounds' Pharmacological Profiles, *in vivo* Targets, Thermoeffectors Recruited and Implications for Drug Development. *Acta Physiologica (Oxford)* 223:e13038 (2018)

35. Brown W, Leff RL, Griffin A, *et al.* Safety, Pharmacokinetics, and Pharmacodynamics Study in Healthy Subjects of Oral NEO6860, a Modality Selective Transient Receptor Potential Vanilloid Subtype 1 Antagonist. *Journal of Pain* 18:726-738 (2017)

36. neomed.ca/en/neomed-therapeutics/therapeutic-projects/Neomed Website. Accessed June 14, 2019.

37. Arsenault P, Leff R, Katz N, *et al.* Analgesic Potential of NEO6860, a Modality Selective TRPV1 Antagonist, in Osteoarthritic Knee Pain: Results of a Randomized, Controlled, Proof-of-Concept Trial. *Arthritis and Rheumatology* 69 (supplement 10): Abstract 2224 (2017) Presented Nov 7, 2017 at the Annual Meeting of the American College of Rheumatology. https://acrab-stracts.org

38. Kwong K and Carr MJ. Voltage-Gated Sodium Channels. *Current Opinions in Pharmacology* 22:131-139 (2015)

39. de Lera Ruiz M and Kraus RL. Voltage-Gated Sodium Channels: Structure, Function, Pharmacology, and Clinical Indications. *Journal of Medicinal Chemistry* 58:7093-7118 (2015)

40. Drenth JPH and Waxman SG. Mutations in Sodium Channel Gene *SCN9A* Cause a Spectrum of Human Genetic Pain Disorders. *Journal of Clinical Investigation* 117:3603-3609 (2007)

41. Waxman SG. Painful Na-Channelopathies: An Expanding Universe. *Trends in Molecular Medicine* 19:406-409 (2013)

42. Teva and Xenon Press Release. Teva and Xenon Provide Update on TV-45070 Phase 2b Study in Osteoarthritis Pain. July 1, 2015.

43. Teva and Xenon Press Release. Teva and Xenon Announce Phase II Study of Topical TV-45070 in Patients with Post-Herpetic Neuralgia (PHN) Did Not Meet Primary Endpoint. June 27, 2017.

44. Zheng YM, Wang WF, Li YF, *et al.* Enhancing Inactivation Rather than Reducing Activation of Nav1.7 Channels by a Clinically Effective Analgesic CNV1014802. *Acta Pharmacologica Sinica* 39:587-596 (2018)

45. https://www.biogen.com/en_us/research-pipeline/biogen-pipeline.html. Accessed Feb 22, 2019.

46. Kumar V and Mahal BA. NGF—the TrkA to Successful Pain Treatment. *Journal of Pain Research* 5:279-286 (2012)

47. Chang DS, Hsu E, Hoffinger DG, and Cohen SP. Anti-Nerve Growth Factor in Pain Management: Current Evidence. *Journal of Pain Research* 9:373-383 (2016)

48. Lane NE, Schnitzer TJ, Birbara CA, *et al.* Tanezumab for the Treatment of Pain from Osteoarthritis of the Knee. *New England Journal of Medicine* 363:1521-1531 (2010)

49. Schnitzer TJ, Lane NE, Birbara CA, *et al.* Long-Term Open-Label Study of Tanezumab for Moderate to Severe Osteoarthritic Knee Pain. *Osteoarthritis and Cartilage* 19:639-646 (2011)

50. Miller RE, Block JA, and Malfait AM. Nerve Growth Factor (NGF) Blockade for the Management of Osteoarthritis Pain: What Can We Learn from Clinical Trials and Preclinical Models? *Current Opinions in Rheumatology* 29:110-118 (2017)

51. Bannwarth B and Kostine M. Nerve Growth Factor Antagonists: Is the Future of Monoclonal Antibodies Becoming Clearer? *Drugs* 77:1377-1387 (2017)

52. Miller RE, Malfait AM, Block JA. Current Status of Nerve Growth Factor Antibodies for the Treatment of Osteoarthritis Pain. *Clinical and Experimental Rheumatology* 35: 85-87 (2017)

53. Pfizer Press Release. Pfizer and Lilly Announce Top-Line Results From Long-Term Phase 3 Study of Tanezumab in Patients With Osteoarthritis. April 18, 2019.

54. Gardner J. Safety Setback for Pfizer, Lilly Pain Drug Should Have Regeneron and Teva Feeling Nervous. *Biopharmadive*. April 22, 2019.

55. www.Regeneron.com/pipeline. Accessed Jan 27, 2020.

56. Special Report. The Role of Science in Addressing the Opioid Crisis. *New England Journal of Medicine* 377:391-394 (2017)

57. Stanczyk MA and Kandasamy R. Biased Agonism: The Quest for the Analgesic Holy Grail. *PAIN Reports* 3:e650 (2018)

58. Ok HG, Kim SY, Lee SJ, *et al.* Can Oliceridine (TRV130), an Ideal Novel μ Receptor G Protein Pathway Selective (μ-GPS) Modulator, Provide Analgesia Without Opioid-Related Adverse Reactions? *Korean Journal of Pain* 31:73-79 (2018)

59. Viscusi ER, Webster L, Kuss M, *et al.* A Randomized, Phase 2 Study Investigating TRV130, a Biased Ligand of the μ-Opioid Receptor for the Intravenous Treatment of Acute Pain. *Pain* 157:264-272 (2016)

60. Presentation to the FDA Advisory Committee. Oliceridine. Meeting of the Anesthetic and Analgesic Drug Products Advisory Committee. Oct 11, 2018.

61. Al Idrus A. FDA Rejects Trevena's Painkiller Oliceridine. *Fierce Biotech*. Nov 5, 2018.

62. Trevena Press Release. Trevena Announces Publication of Results from Phase 3 "Real World" Safety Study for Oliceridine in the *Journal of Pain Research*. Nov 20, 2019.

63. Manglik A, Lin H, Aryal DK, *et al.* Structure-Based Discovery of Opioid Analgesics with Reduced Side Effects. *Nature* 537:185-190 (2016)

64. Rood J. The Quest for Safer Opioid Drugs. *The Scientist Magazine.* Jan 1, 2018.

65. Corder G, Ahanonu B, Grewe BF, *et al.* An Amygdalar Neural Ensemble that Encodes the Unpleasantness of Pain. *Science* 363:276-281 (2019)

66. Lambert J. Scientists Find Brain Cells that Make Pain Hurt. *National Public Radio.* Jan *17, 2019.*

67. Yekkirala AS, Roberson DP, Bean BP and Woolf CJ. Breaking Barriers to Novel Analgesic Drug Development. *Nature Reviews Drug Discovery* 16:545-564 (2017)

68. Kennedy EM. Concession Speech in Campaign for Nomination as the Democratic Presidential Candidate. (1980)

Chapter 9.

1. Cherkin DC and Herman PM. Cognitive and Mind-Body Therapies for Chronic Low Back Pain and Neck Pain. Effectiveness and Value. *JAMA Internal Medicine* 178: 556-557 (2018)

2. Harrison L. Spinal Manipulation for Back and Neck Pain: Does It Work? *Medscape*. Feb 15, 2017.

3. Paige NM, Miake-Lye IM, Booth MS, *et al.* Association of Spinal Manipulative Therapy with Clinical Benefit and Harm for Acute Low Back Pain. Systematic Review and Meta-analysis. *Journal of the American Medical Association* 317:1451-1460 (2017)

4. Deyo RA. Editorial. The Role of Spinal Manipulation in the Treatment of Low Back Pain. *Journal of the American Medical Association* 317:1418-1419 (2017)

5. Goertz CM, Long CR, Vining RD*, et al.* Effect of Usual Medical Care Plus Chiropractic Care vs Usual Medical Care Alone on Pain and Disability Among US Service members with Low Back Pain. A Comparative Effectiveness Clinical Trial. *JAMA Network Open.* e180105.doi.10.1001 (2018)

6. Wheeler AH, Berman SA, Schneck MJ, *et al.* Low Back Pain and Sciatica. *Medscape Reference. Drugs, Diseases and Procedures.* Jan 8, 2013.

7. Standaert CJ, Friedly J, Erwin MW, *et al.* Comparative Effectiveness of Exercise, Acupuncture and Spinal Manipulation for Low Back Pain. *Spine* 36: S120-S130 (2011)

8. Eleswarapu AS, Divi SN, Dirschl DR, *et al.* How Effective Is Physical Therapy for Common Low Back Pain Diagnoses? *Spine* 41:1325-1329 (2016)

9. Cooper G. *Acupuncture for Musculoskeletal Medicine.* Philadelphia. Wolters Kluwer Health/Lippincott Williams & Wilkins (2009)

10. Reston J. Now, About My Operation in Peking. *New York Times.* July 25, 1971.

11. Harrison L. Acupuncture Causes Brain Changes in Patients With Hand Pain. *Medscape.* May 28, 2015.

12. Maeda Y, Kettner N, Kim J, *et al.* Cortical Thickness Increase Following Acupuncture Therapy Is Associated with Symptom Improvement in Idiopathic Hand Pain. *Journal of Pain* 16: Abstract #536 (2015) Poster presentation at the American Pain Society Meeting May 2015.

13. Gozani SN. Science Behind Quell™ Wearable Pain Relief Technology for Treatment of Chronic Pain. PN2204114 Rev. B. NeuroMetrix, Inc. (2015)

14. Gozani SN. Fixed-Site High-Frequency Transcutaneous Electrical Nerve Stimulation for Treatment of Chronic Low Back and Lower Extremity Pain. *Journal of Pain Research* 9:469-479 (2016)

15. Harrison P. Scrambler Therapy Benefit in Cancer-Related Neuropathic Pain. *Medscape*. Jan 11, 2016.

16. Pachman DR, Weisbrod BL, Seisler DK, *et al*. Pilot Evaluation of Scrambler Therapy for the Treatment of Chemotherapy-Induced Peripheral Neuropathy. *Support Care Cancer* 23:943-951 (2015)

17. Khedr EM, Kotb H, Kamel NF, *et al*. Longlasting Antalgic Effects of Daily Sessions of Repetitive Transcranial Magnetic Stimulation in Central and Peripheral Neuropathic Pain. *Journal of Neurology, Neurosurgery, and Psychiatry* 76: 833-838 (2005)

18. Leung A, Donohue M, Xu R, *et al*. rTMS for Suppressing Neuropathic Pain: A Meta-Analysis. *Journal of Pain* 10:1205-1216 (2009)

19. Wysong PB. Successes and Snags in Brain Stimulation for Pain. *Medscape*. Aug 5, 2016.

20. Cameron T. Safety and Efficacy of Spinal Cord Stimulation for the Treatment of Chronic Pain: A 20-Year Literature Review. *Journal of Neurosurgery: Spine* 100:254-267 (2004)

21. Geurts JW, Joosten EA, and van Kleef M. Current Status and Future Perspectives of Spinal Cord Stimulation in Treatment of Chronic Pain. *Pain* 158: 771-774 (2017)

22. Anderson P. Spinal Cord Stimulation Beats Medication for Pain. *Medscape*. May 2, 2018. Discusses information presented by Dr. Tim Lamer at the 2018 annual meeting of the American Academy of Pain Medicine. Abstract LB002. Presented April 27, 2018.

23. van Beek M, Geurts JW, Slangen R, *et al*. Severity of Neuropathy is Associated with Long-Term Spinal Cord Stimulation Outcome in Painful Diabetic Peripheral Neuropathy: Five-Year Follow-Up of a Prospective Two-Center Clinical Trial. *Diabetes Care* 41:32-38 (2018)

24. Medtronic Press Release. Medtronic Announes FDA Clearance and U.S. Launch of the Accurian Radio Frequency System for Nerve Tissue Ablation. Feb 27, 2019.

25. Andrews M. Holistic Therapy Programs May Help Pain Sufferers Ditch Opioids. *National Public Radio*. Aug 29, 2017.

26. Fordyce W. *Behavioral Methods for Chronic Pain and Illness*. Mosby. St. Louis (1976)

27. Main CJ, Keefe FJ, Jensen MP, *et al.* (eds.) *Fordyce's Behavioral Methods for Chronic Pain and Illness: Republished with Invited Commentaries.* Wolters Kluwer Health. Philadelphia (2015)

28. Turk DC, Meichenbaum D, and Genest M. *Pain and Behavioral Medicine: A Cognitive-Behavioral Perspective.* The Guilford Press. New York; London (1983)

29. Brena SF. *Pain and Religion: A Psychophysiologic Study.* Thomas. Springfield, IL (1972)

30. Brena SF. Mental Disorders and Pain. pp. 130-132. In *Pain and Religion: A Psychophysiologic Study.* Thomas. Springfield, IL (1972)

31. Majeed MH, Sudak DM. Cognitive Behavioral Therapy for Chronic Pain – One Therapeutic Approach for the Opioid Epidemic. *Journal of Psychiatric Practice* 23:409-414 (2017)

32. Swift Yasgur B, Barclay L. Role of CBT in the Treatment of Chronic Pain. *Medscape.* Jan 26, 2018.

33. Marchant J. A Placebo Treatment for Pain. *New York Times.* Jan 10, 2016.

34. Akil H. The Dawn of Endorphins. pp. 99-110 In *Opioids and Pain Relief: A Historical Perspective* Meldrum ML (ed.) IASP Press. Seattle (2003)

35. Colloca L, Klinger R, Flor H, and Bingel U. Placebo Analgesia: Psychological and Neurobiological Mechanisms. *Pain* 154:511-514 (2013)

36. Diederich NJ and Goetz CA. The Placebo Treatments in Neurosciences. New Insights from Clinical and Neuroimaging Studies. *Neurology* 71:677-684 (2008)

37. Wager TD, Rilling JK, Smith EE, *et al.* Placebo-Induced Changes in fMRI in the Anticipation and Experience of Pain. *Science* 303:1162-1167(2004)

38. Petrovic P, Kalso, E, Petersson KM, and Ingvar M. Placebo and Opioid Analgesia – Imaging a Shared Neuronal Network. *Science* 295:1737-1740 (2002)

39. Goffaux P, Redmond WJ, Rainville P and Marchand S. Descending Analgesia – When the Spine Echoes What the Brain Expects. *Pain* 130:137-143 (2007)

40. Zunhammer M, Bingel U, and Wager TD. Placebo Effects on the Neurologic Pain Signature. A Meta-Analysis of Individual Participant Functional Magnetic Resonance Imaging Data. *JAMA Neurology.* Published online July 30, 2018.

41. Cahana A and Romagnioli S. Not All Placebos Are the Same: A Debate on the Ethics of Placebo Use in Clinical Trials Versus Clinical Practice. *Journal of Anesthesiology* 21:102-105 (2007)

42. Kisaalita N, Staud R, Hurley R, and Robinson M. Placebo Use in Pain Management: The Role of Medical Context, Treatment Efficacy, and Deception in Determining Placebo Acceptability. *Pain* 155:2638-2645 (2014)
43. Zeidan F, Emerson NM, Farris SR, *et al.* Mindfulness Meditation-Based Pain Relief Employs Different Neural Mechanisms Than Placebo and Sham Mindfulness Meditation-Induced Analgesia. *Journal of Neuroscience* 35:15307-15325 (2015)

Chapter 10.

1. Bao Y, Pan Y, Taylor A, *et al.* Prescription Drug Monitoring Programs are Associated with Sustained Reductions in Opioid Prescribing by Physicians. *Health Affairs* 35:1045-1051 (2016)
2. Coffin PO, Behar E, Rowe C, *et al.* Nonrandomized Intervention Study of Naloxone Co-prescription for Primary Care Patients Receiving Long-Term Opioid Therapy for Pain. *Annals of Internal Medicine* 165:245-252 (2016)
3. White House Press Release. FACT SHEET: Obama Administration Announces Additional Actions to Address the Prescription Opioid Abuse and Heroin Epidemic. March 28, 2016.
4. Hensley, S. Poll: Most Americans Know About Opioid Antidote and Are Willing to Use It. *National Public Radio.* August 21, 2018.
5. Harper J. Reversing an Overdose Isn't Complicated, But Getting the Antidote Can Be. *National Public Radio*. May 7, 2018.
6. Feder Ostrov B. More States Say Doctors Must Offer Naloxone Along with Opioids. *Medscape*. Feb 21, 2019.
7. Beletsky L. With Advent of EVZIO for Lay Reversal of Opioid Overdose, Enthusiasm and Caution. *American Journal of Preventive Medicine* 48:357-359 (2015)
8. Gupta R, Shah ND and Ross JS. The Rising Price of Naloxone - Risks to Efforts to Stem Overdose Deaths. *New England Journal of Medicine* 375: 2213-2215 (2016)
9. Kaléo Press Release. Authorized Generic for EVZIO™ (naloxone injection). Dec 12, 2018.
10. Schatman ME. The Role of the Health Insurance Industry in Perpetuating Suboptimal Pain Management. *Pain Medicine* 12: 415-426 (2011)
11. Heyward J, Jones CM, Compton WM, *et al.* Coverage of Nonpharmacologic Treatments for Low Back Pain Among US Public and Private Insurers. *JAMA*

Network Open. 2018; 1(6): e183044.doi:10.1001/jamanetworkopen. 2018.3044

12. Petersen KL and Rowbotham MC. Quantitative Sensory Testing Scaled Up for Multicenter Clinical Research Networks: A Promising Start. *Pain* 123:219-220 (2006)

13. Chizh BA, Priestley T, Rowbotham M and Schaffler K. Predicting Therapeutic Efficacy – Experimental Pain in Human Subjects. *Brain Research Reviews* 60:243-254 (2009)

14. Kosek E, Ekholm J and Hansson P. Sensory Dysfunction in Fibromyalgia Patients with Implications for Pathogenic Mechanisms. *Pain* 68:375-383 (1996)

15. Borsook D, Moulton EA, Schmidt KF and Becerra LR. Neuroimaging Revolutionizes Therapeutic Approaches to Chronic Pain. *Molecular Pain* 3:25-32 (2007)

16. May, A. Structural Brain Imaging: A Window into Chronic Pain. *The Neuroscientist* 17:209-220 (2011)

17. Baliki MN, Schnitzer TJ, Bauer WR, and Apkarian AV. Brain Morphological Signatures for Chronic Pain. *PLoS One* 6:e26010 (2011)

18. Ung H, Brown JE, Johnson KA, *et al.* Multivariate Classification of Structural MRI Data Detects Chronic Low Back Pain. *Cerebral Cortex* 24: 1037-1044 (2014)

19. Martucci KT, Ng P, and Mackey S. Neuroimaging Chronic Pain: What Have We Learned and Where Are We Going? *Future Neurology* 9:615-626 (2014)

20. Kuchinad A, Schweinhardt P, Seminowicz DA, *et al.* Accelerated Brain Gray Matter Loss in Fibromyalgia Patients: Premature Aging of the Brain? *Journal of Neuroscience* 27:4004-4007 (2007)

21. Robinson ME, Craggs JG, Price DD, *et al.* Gray Matter Volumes of Pain-Related Brain Areas Are Decreased in Fibromyalgia Syndrome. *Journal of Pain* 12:436-443 (2011)

22. Apkarian AV, Sosa Y, Sonty S, *et al.* Chronic Back Pain Is Associated with Decreased Prefrontal and Thalamic Gray Matter Density. *Journal of Neuroscience* 24:10410-10415 (2004)

23. Hashmi JA, Baliki MN, Huang L, *et al.* Shape Shifting Pain: Chronification of Back Pain Shifts Brain Representation from Nociceptive to Emotional Circuits. *Brain* 136:2751-2768 (2013)

24. Seminowicz DA, Wideman TH, Naso L, *et al.* Effective Treatment of Chronic Low Back Pain in Humans Reverses Abnormal Brain Anatomy and Function. *Journal of Neuroscience* 31:7540-7550 (2011)

25. Gwilym SE, Filippini N, Douaud G, *et al*. Thalamic Atrophy Associated with Painful Osteoarthritis of the Hip is Reversible After Arthroplasty: A Longitudinal Voxel-Based Morphometric Study. *Arthritis and Rheumat*ism 62:2930-2940 (2010)

26. Tracey I. Taking the Narrative Out of Pain: Objectifying Pain Through Brain Imaging. Chapter 9. pp. 127-163. In *Narrative, Pain and Suffering*. Carr DB, Loeser JD and Morris DB (eds.) IASP Press. Seattle (2005)

27. Wager TD, Atlas LY, Lindquist MA, *et al*. An fMRI-Based Neurologic Signature of Physical Pain. *New England Journal of Medicine* 368:1388-1397 (2013)

28. Williams DA and Clauw DJ. Understanding Fibromyalgia: Lessons from the Broader Pain Research Community. *Journal of Pain* 10: 777-791 (2009)

29. Jensen KB, Kosek E, Petzke F, *et al*. Evidence of Dysfunctional Pain Inhibition in Fibromyalgia Reflected in rACC During Provoked Pain. *Pain* 144: 95-100 (2009)

30. Staud R. Brain Imaging in Fibromyalgia Syndrome. *Clinical and Experimental Rheumatology* 29 (suppl 69): 109-117 (2011)

31. Jensen KB, Srinivasan P, Spaeth R, *et al*. Overlapping Structural and Functional Brain Changes in Patients with Long-Term Exposure to Fibromyalgia Pain. *Arthritis and Rheumat*ism 65: 3293-3303 (2013)

32. Cagnie B, Coppieters I, Denecker S, *et al*. Central Sensitization in Fibromyalgia? A Systematic Review on Structural and Functional Brain MRI. *Seminars in Arthritis and Rheumatism* 44:68-75 (2014)

33. Lopez-Sola M, Woo C-W, Pujol J, *et al*. Towards a Neurophysiological Signature for Fibromyalgia. *Pain* 158:34-37 (2017)

34. Baliki MN, Chiavlo DR, Geha PY, *et al*. Chronic Pain and the Emotional Brain: Specific Brain Activity Associated with Spontaneous Fluctuations of Intensity of Chronic Back Pain. *Journal of Neuroscience* 26:12165-12173 (2006)

35. Geha PY, Baliki MN, Chialvo DR, *et al*. Brain Activity for Spontaneous Pain of Post-Herpetic Neuralgia and Its Modulation by Lidocaine Patch Therapy. *Pain* 128: 88-100 (2007)

36. Borsook D, Becerra L, and Hargreaves R. Biomarkers for Chronic Pain and Analgesia. Part 1: The Need, Reality, Challenges, and Solutions. *Discovery Medicine* 11:197-207 (2011)

37. Borsook D, Becerra L, and Hargreaves R. Biomarkers for Chronic Pain and Analgesia. Part 2: How, Where, and What to Look for Using Functional Imaging. *Discovery Medicine* 11:209-219 (2011)

38. Twilley N. Seeing Pain. *The New Yorker*. July 2, 2018.

39. Tian Y, Liu X, Jia M, *et al.* Targeted Genotyping Identifies Susceptibility Locus in Brain-Derived Neurotrophic Factor Gene for Chronic Postsurgical Pain. *Anesthesiology* 128: 587-597 (2018)

40. Correia MA. Drug Biotransformation. Chapter 4. pp. 53-68. In *Basic and Clinical Pharmacology*. 12th edition. Katzung BG, Masters SB, and Trevor AJ (eds.) McGraw Hill. New York (2012)

41. Singa RM. Genetic Testing: Adjunct in the Medical Management of Chronic Pain. *Practical Pain Management*. Vol 16. Issue 4. May 2016.

42. Anderson P. Have Difficult-to-Treat Pain Patients? Try Genetic Testing. *Medscape*. March 2, 2016.

43. Zahari Z and Ismail R. Influence of Cytochrome P450, Family 2, Subfamily D, Polypeptide 6 (*CYP2D6*) Polymorphisms on Pain Sensitivity and Clinical Response to Weak Opioid Analgesics. *Drug Metabolism and Pharmacokinetics* 29:29-43 (2014)

44. Miotto K, Cho AK, Khalil MA, *et al.* Trends in Tramadol: Pharmacology, Metabolism, and Misuse. *Anesthesia and Analgesia* 124: 44-51 (2017)

45. Gaedigk A, Bhathena A, Ndjountche L, *et al.* Identification and Characterization of Novel Sequence Variations in the Cytochrome P4502D6 (*CYP2D6*) Gene in African Americans. *Pharmacogenomics Journal* 5:173-182 (2005)

46. Rodieux F, Pigeut V, Berney B, *et al.* Pharmacogenetics and Analgesic Effects of Antidepressants in Chronic Pain Management. *Personalized Medicine* 12:163-175 (2015)

47. CYP2D6 Genotyping. https://www.genelex.com/test-menu/CYP2D6

48. Farmer B. Nashville Public Radio. Amid Opioid Prescriber Crackdown, Officials Reach Out to Pain Patients. *Medscape*. April 30, 2019.

49. Melville NA. Landmark Surgeon General Report Tackles Addiction. *Medscape.* Nov 18, 2016. Report entitled "Facing Addiction in America: The Surgeon General's Report on Alcohol, Drugs, and Health"

50. Califf RM, Woodcock J and Ostroff S. A Proactive Response to Prescription Opioid Abuse. *New England Journal of Medicine* 374:1480-1485 (2016)

51. Strict Rules Hinder Addiction Treatment. Editorial. *New York Times*. March 27, 2019.

52. Young KD. Stop Limiting Access to Opioid Addiction Meds, Experts Say. *Medscape*. March 22, 2019.

53. Bruehl S, Apkarian AV, Ballantyne JC, *et al.* Personalized Medicine and Opioid Analgesic Prescribing for Chronic Pain: Opportunities and Challenges. *Journal of Pain* 14:103-113 (2013)

INDEX

CPSIA information can be obtained
at www.ICGtesting.com
Printed in the USA
BVHW040013140520
579671BV00012B/180/J